WITHDRAWN

HYPERPARATHYROIDISM

Publication Number 173
AMERICAN LECTURE SERIES®

A *Monograph in*
AMERICAN LECTURES IN ENDOCRINOLOGY

Edited by
WILLARD O. THOMPSON, M.D.
Clinical Professor of Medicine
University of Illinois College of Medicine
Managing Editor, Journal of Clinical Endocrinology and Metabolism
Editor, Journal of the American Geriatrics Society
Chicago, Illinois

HYPERPARATHYROIDISM

By

B. MARDEN BLACK, M.D.

Associate Professor of Surgery
Mayo Foundation for Medical Education and Research
Graduate School, University of Minnesota
and
Division of Surgery
Mayo Clinic
Rochester, Minnesota

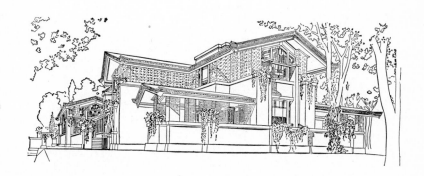

CHARLES C THOMAS · PUBLISHER

Springfield · Illinois · U.S.A.

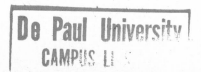

CHARLES C THOMAS · PUBLISHER
BANNERSTONE HOUSE
301-327 EAST LAWRENCE AVENUE, SPRINGFIELD, ILLINOIS, U.S.A.

Published simultaneously in the British Commonwealth of Nations by
BLACKWELL SCIENTIFIC PUBLICATIONS, LTD., OXFORD, ENGLAND

Published simultaneously in Canada by
THE RYERSON PRESS, TORONTO

Library of Congress Catalog Card Number: 53-8630

Printed in the United States of America

CONTENTS

Chapter

HYPERPARATHYROIDISM

Chapter *I*

INTRODUCTION

H YPERPARATHYROIDISM is a relatively common, potentially fatal disease which, if treated before irreversible renal damage has been produced, is curable in the great majority of cases. Neither the diagnosis nor the treatment is particularly difficult. A working knowledge of the disease, as it is known at present, evolved some 15 to 20 years ago. Failure to apply this knowledge clinically is responsible for the fact that hyperparathyroidism is still widely regarded as a rare disease of little general interest or importance. It was because of the belief that the condition is still being largely overlooked, and that another review of the subject might broaden interest in hyperparathyroidism, that I rather welcomed the opportunity to contribute the volume on hyperparathyroidism to the *American Lecture Series.*

An attempt has been made to assemble the information necessary to diagnose and treat hyperparathyroidism successfully. It should be emphasized, however, that successful case-finding and treatment demand a special interest on the part of internist, roentgenologist, clinical pathologist, tissue pathologist and surgeon. The number of cases found will depend to a large extent on how regularly calcium determinations are carried out in cases of urinary lithiasis, so that the urologist becomes a most important member of the group. Unless there is a joint interest in hyperparathyroidism, the diagnosis is likely to be uncertain and rarely made, while treatment will be largely unsatisfactory.

As a basis for the review, I have drawn heavily on the

3

Mayo Clinic series of proved cases, which numbered 112 through 1949. The series is sufficiently large to include most of the variables which might be expected in the study of any disease. It is probably also more representative than the cases reported in the literature, since the reported series is still weighted unduly with cases of generalized osteitis fibrosa. For obvious reasons, only proved cases have been included in the series.

I would like to take this opportunity to express my appreciation and thanks to the members of the Section on Metabolic Disease of the Mayo Clinic, particularly to Dr. F. R. Keating, Jr., for many suggestions concerning the clinical aspects; to Dr. L. B. Woolner, of the Division of Surgical Pathology, who has recently reviewed all pathologic material pertaining to cases of hyperparathyroidism in our series; and to Dr. D. G. Pugh, of the Section of Roentgenology, for his assistance in clarifying the roentgenologic aspects. Finally, any review of hyperparathyroidism would be incomplete without specifically recognizing the contributions to the subject of Dr. Fuller Albright and his colleagues, which have largely made possible the present understanding of the disease.

Chapter II

HISTORICAL

THE SKELETAL disease caused by hyperparathyroidism was clearly described by von Recklinghausen in 1891. Among a group of 16 necropsy cases of osseous disease there were three in which the bony changes were very similar if not identical to generalized osteitis fibrosa, and Case 7 was certainly an example of the osseous disease caused by hyperparathyroidism. In this case, extensive fibrosis, cysts, and brown tumors were emphasized, and the patient had had many spontaneous fractures. The etiology of the disease was not suspected nor was even the existence of the parathyroid glands, although they had been discovered 11 years previously. Sandstrom (1880) not only described the four parathyroid glands but illustrated correctly their relationship to the thyroid (Fig. 1). He expressed some amazement that such definite and constant structures had not been recognized previously. His discovery went quite unnoticed. It was not until the riddle of post-thyroidectomy tetany and myxedema was being unraveled that the parathyroids were again recognized. Gley (1891) rediscovered the external parathyroids and Kohn (1895) the so-called internal pair. The relationship of the glands to tetany was finally proved by ablation experiments by Vassale and Generali in 1900.

The first report of the association of a parathyroid tumor and generalized osteitis fibrosa was made by Askanazy in 1904. The case was that of a woman, aged 51 years, who had severe pains in the extremities and many spontaneous fractures. At necropsy the osseous disease was recognized as that which had been described by von Reckling-

5

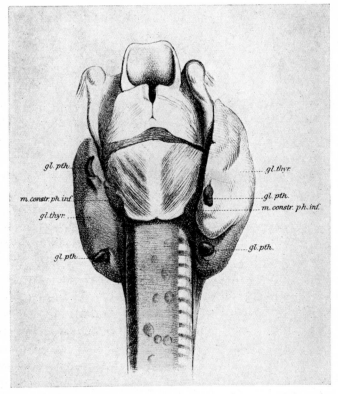

FIG 1. The illustration which accompanied the original description of the parathyroid glands by Sandstrom. The positions of the four glands and their relationship to the thyroid are shown beautifully.

hausen, and a tumor was found lateral to the left lobe of the thyroid. The tumor was not emphasized nor was its significance recognized, although it was suspected of being of parathyroid origin. The fundamental step of associating osseous disease with enlargement of the parathyroid glands was made by Erdheim in 1907. He had noted the year previously that calcification of the incisor teeth of rats became faulty after destruction of the parathyroid glands. This observation led to studies of the parathyroid glands at necropsy in cases of osteomalacia. In 1907, he described three cases of osteomalacia in which the parathyroid glands were hyperplastic. His report attracted wide attention, and other similar cases were soon described. By 1925, Hoffheinz was able to collect from the literature data on 45 cases in which measurable enlargement of the parathyroid glands had been found at necropsy. Skeletal disease was associated with the parathyroid enlargement in 27 of the 45 cases. Seventeen were cases of generalized osteitis fibrosa, eight of osteomalacia and two of rickets.

The observation that calcification of the rat's incisor teeth became faulty after destruction of the parathyroids, together with the finding of hyperplasia of the parathyroids at necropsy in cases of osteomalacia and rickets, led Erdheim to the conclusion that the changes in the parathyroids were compensatory in character and consequently were the result rather than the cause of the osseous disease. Erdheim's views concerning the relationship of changes in the parathyroids to the osseous disease have long been considered to have delayed the surgical treatment of generalized osteitis fibrosa. Albright[4] (1948) has recently set the record straight in this respect. He pointed out that in rickets and osteomalacia there is indeed hyperplasia of the parathyroid glands and that the hyperplasia is compensatory in character. In short, Erdheim's conclusions were perfectly sound. According to Albright, Erdheim was not opposed to parathyroidectomy in cases of generalized osteitis fibrosa and, in fact, never expressed himself concerning the question.

Nevertheless, the view was current prior to 1925 that the changes in the parathyroid glands in cases of generalized osteitis fibrosa were compensatory and not the cause

of the osseous disease. This conception was first chal-
lenged in 1915 by Schlagenhaufer, who pointed out that
in many cases of osseous disease with associated changes
in the parathyroids one gland only was enlarged. He
reasoned that this would be difficult to explain if the enlargements were compensatory. He concluded that the
enlarged parathyroid might well be the cause of the
osseous disease and that parathyroidectomy might be
beneficial in certain cases of malacic disease of bone. According to Shelling the proposal was rejected by Bauer,
a surgeon, on the grounds that it was too radical and too
dangerous.[102]

In 1925, about 10 years after Schlagenhaufer's proposal, Mandl[78] carried out the first parathyroidectomy during life. The events leading to the exploration of the parathyroids and the outcome of the case are of considerable
historic interest and importance. The patient was a pen-
sioned streetcar conductor aged 38 years. Generalized
osteitis fibrosa had developed four years before the operation, and the correct diagnosis had been established roentgenographically two years later. In keeping with the then
current views that the skeletal disease was primary, treatment with cod-liver oil was tried, but without benefit. An
extract of the parathyroid glands of animals was next tried,
again without affecting the disease. Mandl then trans-
planted the parathyroid glands, removed from a person
who was moribund as the result of an accident, into the
abdominal wall of the patient. He became convinced that
this made the patient worse rather than better as had been
anticipated, and on this basis, the decision was made to
explore the parathyroids. The tumor, an adenoma of the
wasserhelle cell type which measured 2.5 by 1.5 by 1.2 cm.,
was found and removed without difficulty.

Improvement after the operation was immediate and

striking. The concentration of calcium in the urine dropped to a fraction of its former value. The pains in the extremities began to improve within a few weeks. The patient was ambulatory on crutches within three months, and definite roentgenologic evidence of recalcification of the skeleton had appeared by this time. Rather ironically, since the case proved conclusively the etiologic relationship of the adenoma to generalized osteitis fibrosa, the improvement did not continue. The bones failed to regain their normal density and the hypercalcemia persisted. Seven years after the first operation, a second cervical exploration was carried out because of an increase in the skeletal lesions and because of renal stones. As is so often the case in secondary operations, no abnormal tissue could be found.[79]

The report of Mandl's case appeared[78] in 1926. The dramatic improvement after the parathyroidectomy served to renew interest in generalized osteitis fibrosa so that a greatly increased number of cases were soon reported. The first case in which successful treatment was accomplished in the United States was reported in 1929 by Barr, Bulger and Dixon, who first proposed the use of the term "hyperparathyroidism" to designate the condition. They pointed out that "in the literature on osteomalacia, on multiple cystic tumors of bone and on parathyroid tumors, there is a clinical picture, found occasionally under all of these titles, which seems to deserve description as a separate clinical entity—as definite and distinct as parathyroid tetany or exophthalmic goiter." Between 1926 and 1934 more than 100 parathyroidectomies were carried out for generalized osteitis fibrosa.[102] These many cases added little to the fundamental knowledge of hyperparathyroidism but tended to fix, instead, the association of generalized osteitis fibrosa and hyperparathyroidism to the point

that the terms became virtually synonymous. The diagnosis of hyperparathyroidism was not made in the absence
of generalized osteitis fibrosa, and roentgenologic changes
along with biopsies of bone were the only methods by
which the diagnosis could be established with certainty.

Developments in the field far more important than the
mere accumulation of cases were meanwhile occurring.
Parathyroid extract was prepared independently by Hanson (1925) and by Collip[35] (1925). Within the next year,
particularly in the laboratories of Collip[35-37] and of Greenwald and Gross, the principal actions of the hormone had
been elucidated. These experimental findings were first
applied clinically in a case of generalized osteitis fibrosa
by Hannon, Shorr, McClellan and DuBois in 1926. Hypercalcemia and hypophosphatemia were demonstrated. Calcium balance studies were carried out, and an intake of
700 mg. of calcium a day was found necessary to equal the
calcium lost by the patient. Treatment by means of parathyroid extract was tried, and this made the patient more
uncomfortable. It was concluded that the patient's disease
agreed in all essentials with the condition produced experimentally in animals by excessive administration of
parathyroid extract. The metabolic changes of the patient
were roughly equivalent to those produced in a normal
person by the administration of 100 units of parathyroid
extract daily.[90] Incidentally, the skeletal disease was not
recognized roentgenologically, indicating how little was
known of generalized osteitis fibrosa at that time in the
United States. It will be recalled that the correct roentgenographic diagnosis had been made in Mandl's case in
1923 in Vienna. Cervical exploration was carried out in
May, 1926, but no tumor was found.[90]

The now famous case of Captain Charles Martell will
not be again reviewed except to mention that the tumor

was not found until the seventh operation and that death due to renal complications occurred a few weeks later. This historic and tragic case is associated with an impressive lot of "firsts": the first case in which the diagnosis was established by biochemical determinations, the first case of generalized osteitis fibrosa in which mineral balance studies were carried out, the first case in the United States and the second in the world in which the parathyroid glands were explored, and the first case in which the removal of uninvolved parathyroid glands was found not to influence the hyperparathyroidism. The case was not reported in full until 1930.[63] By this time, Gold (1928), Barr, Bulger and Dixon (1929) and Wilder (1929) had each reported data on cases in which biochemical studies had been carried out and in each of which a parathyroid adenoma had been found and removed.

Studies of calcium balance in clinical cases of hyperparathyroidism and experimental studies of the action of parathyroid hormone both emphasized the increased excretion of calcium in the urine. The hypercalciuria of hyperparathyroidism logically suggested the possibility of calcium deposition in the kidneys and lower part of the urinary tract. The association of osseous disease with the renal insufficiency of urinary lithiasis had been occasionally reported previously. Davies-Colley (1884) reported the case of a child aged nine years who had extensive osseous disease and multiple calculi of kidneys and ureters. Hubbard and Wentworth (1921) found at necropsy generalized osteitis fibrosa, nephritis and hyperplasia of the parathyroids. In the case reported by Gaugele (1907) the osseous disease was complicated by infected hydronephrosis caused by stones. Jacoby and Schroth (1912) demonstrated an abnormally high excretion of calcium in the urine in a case of generalized osteitis fibrosa.

MacCallum (1905) first reported the association of a parathyroid tumor and extensive renal disease but no osseous disease. The patient had died of uremia. The parathyroid tumor measured 2 cm. in diameter, and there were no strands of fatty tissue within the parenchyma. The virtual absence of stromal fat is the most striking microscopic feature of a parathyroid adenoma. Mitotic figures "of great beauty" were seen. Mitoses have since been observed repeatedly in parathyroid adenomas. This finding, along with other cytologic changes, has given rise to a still unsettled controversy as to whether the usual parathyroid tumor is malignant or benign. By 1934 Gutman, Swenson and Parsons were able to find reports of 112 cases of proved hyperparathyroidism in the literature. Renal colics had occurred in 10 per cent of the reported cases.

It was not, however, until the paper of Albright, Aub and Bauer (1934) that the importance of the renal complications was fully appreciated. By presenting data on 17 proved cases from one institution, in 11 of which the diagnosis had been made at the Massachusetts General Hospital, they demonstrated conclusively that hyperparathyroidism was not particularly uncommon. Urinary calculi were present in 10 of the 17 cases, in seven of which symptoms were limited to those caused by the calculi. In five cases there was no evidence of osseous disease. Hyperparathyroidism was diagnosed in eight of the 17 cases only because determinations of serum calcium and phosphorus had been carried out in cases of urinary lithiasis. In addition to stressing the importance of the urinary complications, and establishing the fact that hyperparathyroidism could occur and be recognized in the absence of generalized osteitis fibrosa, diagnostic criteria were fully described. The prediction, which has been amply verified since,[39] was made that hyperparathyroidism would turn out to be a fairly common cause of urinary stones and that hyperparathyroidism with renal complications would prove more common than generalized osteitis fibrosa.

Advances in the field since 1934 have been those which would be expected to follow the accumulation of increasing numbers of cases. The pathology of hyperparathyroidism was placed on a workable basis by Castleman and Mallory[31] in 1935. The earlier, limited conceptions of surgical treatment expressed by Mandl (1926,[78] 1933[79]) and by Walton (1931) were extended virtually to those of the present by Churchill and Cope (1934), and by Cope[38] (1941). The first hyperfunctioning carcinoma of parathyroid origin with metastasis was reported in 1939.[83] The association of peptic ulcer and hyperparathyroidism was first emphasized by Rogers (1946) and by Rogers, Keating, Morlock and Barker (1947). Of greater importance, since 1934, has been the gradual acceptance of the thesis of the Boston group that hyperparathyroidism must be excluded in all cases of urinary lithiasis.

The importance of this approach to the disease is well illustrated by the experience at the Mayo Clinic. The diagnosis in the first case in the clinic series was proved at operation in December, 1928, probably the second proved case in America. In spite of this early and since continued interest in hyperparathyroidism, an average of one case only was proved each year during the succeeding 12 years. The almost unbelievable success of the Boston group in case-finding occasioned a comprehensive review of the world's literature and of the practices at the Mayo Clinic with respect to hyperparathyroidism by Wilder and Howell in 1936. Two years later, Griffin, Osterberg and Braasch completed a review of more than 1,200 cases of renal lithiasis and found that in two cases only was there an associated hyperparathyroidism. The implied conclusion in both papers was that the condition was exceedingly rare among patients seen at the Mayo Clinic. Five years later, having meanwhile become convinced that the experiences of Albright and his colleagues could be duplicated, internists and urologists at the clinic made a concerted joint effort to establish the diagnosis in more cases. The effect was immediately rewarded by the finding of four cases within less than six months. In the succeeding seven years, the diagnosis was made in more than 90 cases. At present between 15 and 20 cases are being recognized each year at the clinic. The increased success in the recognition of hyperparathyroidism here can be attributed almost entirely to a more careful screening of patients with urinary lithiasis for hypercalcemia. This approach to the problem of finding cases of hyperparathyroidism has yielded two series of cases (Massachusetts General Hospital series; Mayo Clinic series) which together probably equal numerically all other reported cases.

Chapter III

PATHOLOGIC PHYSIOLOGY

HYPERPARATHYROIDISM is characterized by an increase in the level of calcium and a decrease in that of phosphorus* in the serum, and by an increased excretion of both in the urine. The same changes follow the injection of parathyroid extract, and changes in the reverse direction occur when the injections are discontinued, or after removal of a hyperfunctioning parathyroid adenoma. The four changes, while obviously interrelated, do not occur at the same time. After an injection of parathyroid extract there is first an immediate increase in the excretion of phosphorus in the urine. Presumably as a consequence the level of phosphorus in the serum falls, and, as the phosphorus falls, the calcium in the serum rises. The increased excretion of calcium in the urine develops as the calcium in the serum rises, so that several hours may elapse between the development of hyperphosphaturia and of hypercalciuria.[3, 7, 10, 84]

This sequence of changes, together with the fact that the hormone affects the excretion of phosphorus in the urine more profoundly than the level of calcium in the serum, led Albright to postulate that the primary action of parathyroid hormone was on the excretion of phosphorus. The other three changes occur as a consequence and depend on the fact that the calcium and phosphorus ions in body fluids are in equilibrium with the calcium-carbonate calcium-phosphate salts of bone. The solubility product of the ionic calcium and phosphorus in tissue

---

* In keeping with Albright's usage, the term "phosphorus" has been used rather than "inorganic phosphate" or "phosphate" phosphorus.

15

fluids is probably a constant so that, at a constant pH, as the phosphorus falls the calcium rises.

The course of events is described by Albright and Reifenstein as follows:

> The parathyroid hormone in some way affects the phosphate dissolved in body fluids in such a way as to make it more readily excreted by the kidney with a resulting decrease in the serum phosphorus level; this tends to make the body fluids less saturated in regard to whatever equilibrium constant governs the serum calcium and phosphorus values; resorption of the calcium-phosphate salt from the bone resorbing surfaces is thereby increased; there results an elevated serum calcium level together with depressed serum phosphorus level. Once the new state of equilibrium has been reached there would be no further changes if it were not for the fact that the higher serum calcium level leads to an increased calcium excretion in the urine; this loss of calcium in the urine is a factor tending to cause undersaturation of the body fluids again so that unless there is a supply of calcium from the gastrointestinal tract the bones will have to supply the deficit; there will result, therefore, a decrease in the total amount of bone tissue and the bones will become weak. As the bones become weak they will be more subject to stresses and strains; this will stimulate the osteoblasts to lay down more osteoid tissue.

The osteoid tissue in hyperparathyroidism calcifies normally and this acts as a further drain on the calcium and phosphorus in body fluids and hence favors further resorption of bone, and further weakening of the skeleton. The increased metaplasia of bone in generalized osteitis fibrosa is very evident histologically.

It should perhaps be added that the osseous changes of hyperparathyroidism result from an augmentation of the same process which occurs normally. That is, normally there is a constant resorption and reformation of bone initiated by the constant normal loss of calcium and phosphorus in the urine. The resulting tendency toward undersaturation of body fluids is countered by resorption of bone, and new bone is formed because of the resulting weakening of the bone. Both the production of osteoid, the organic matrix of bone, and precipitation of inorganic salts are functions of the osteoblasts. The latter process is enzymatic and occurs because of a local increase of phosphate ions resulting from the action of alkaline phosphatase formed by the osteoblasts. The enzyme acts by splitting inorganic phosphate from organic phosphorus compounds.[92] A second enzyme, phosphorylase, is probably involved to supply the substrate high in organic phosphorus compounds on which the alkaline phosphatase acts.[58] The small amount of alkaline phosphatase normally present in serum is a reflection of this normal osteoblastic activity. Since osteoid calcifies in hyperparathyroidism, it must be assumed that what Albright calls the local calcifying factor (the alkaline phosphatase-phosphorylase mechanism) is sufficient to compensate for the undersaturation of calcium and phosphorus ions in the body fluids.

In addition to causing a phosphate diuresis, the parathyroid hormone has a direct decalcifying action on bone.[70, 81, 101, 105] In nephrectomized animals, a rise in serum calcium has been demonstrated after injection of parathyroid hormone.[44] Ingalls and his colleagues have shown that the action is independent of the acidosis which develops after nephrectomy and of that due to the acidity of the parathyroid extract. Wilton (1946) has proposed that the hormone acts by preventing maturation of the osteoblasts. The immature osteoblasts are presumably unable to produce the enzymes necessary for the precipitation of bone salts.

Clinical experience with hyperparathyroidism suggests strongly that the phosphate diuresis is more important than the direct decalcification of bone, since even fairly severe hyperparathyroidism may exist without demonstrable evidence of skeletal disease. Furthermore, it is now generally accepted that if the intake of calcium is sufficiently high to maintain a positive calcium balance in hyperparathyroidism, skeletal disease will not develop. If the hormone acted predominantly to increase the dissolution of osseous tissue directly, the most common clinical form of the disease, that is, hyperparathyroidism without osseous disease, would be difficult to explain, particularly since the value for alkaline phosphatase is normal in such cases.

The formation of parathyroid hormone is presumably governed by the level of ionic calcium in the serum. In conditions in which the level of calcium tends to be low, such as osteomalacia, the parathyroid glands become hypertrophied and hyperplastic.[9] Conversely, in conditions in which the ionic calcium is increased, for example, hyperparathyroidism due to an adenoma, the uninvolved glands are atrophic. The reciprocal relationship between the levels of ionic calcium and phosphorus in the serum, as well as the primary action of the hormone on the excretion of phosphorus, suggests the possibility that an increase in the level of phosphorus in the serum might act as a stimulus for the production of hormone. Crawford and associates (1950) have recently published experimental data supporting this conception. It seems probable, therefore, that both a decrease in the level of calcium and an increase in that of phosphorus act as a stimulus to the parathyroid glands.

The possibility of a parathyrotropic pituitary factor has been investigated extensively. The evidence is, on the whole, conflicting. Engfeldt (1950), after an extensive reinvestigation of the problem, concluded that there was no such factor in the anterior lobe of the pituitary. He found, however, that the level of phosphorus declined after hypophysectomy provided that the adrenals were intact, suggesting an indirect action of the pituitary on the parathyroids.

Chapter IV

PATHOLOGY

Primary hyperparathyroidism may be caused by a single adenoma, by multiple adenomas, by primary (wasserhelle) hyperplasia or by carcinoma. The incidence of the different lesions in the Mayo Clinic series is shown in Table I. If the series is representative, a single adenoma may be expected in approximately 80 per cent of cases;

TABLE I. GROSS PATHOLOGY: 112 CASES
OF PROVED HYPERPARATHYROIDISM

Single adenoma	92
Multiple adenomas	10
Primary (wasserhelle) hyperplasia	9
Carcinoma with metastasis	1

multiple adenomas, involving more than one parathyroid gland, in 10 per cent; and primary hyperplasia in the remaining 10 per cent. Hyperfunctioning carcinoma is fortunately rare, accounting for probably not more than 1 or 2 per cent of cases.

SINGLE ADENOMA

Parathyroid adenomas vary in weight from 30 to 40 mg., the weight of a normal parathyroid gland, to 100 gm. or even more. A remnant of normal parathyroid tissue may occasionally be found just outside of the capsule of smaller adenomas, or a small appendage of normal parathyroid tissue may be attached to the capsule of the adenoma (Fig. 2). The form of the adenoma is largely dependent on neighboring structures. Small tumors tend to be caught in sulci of the thyroid or between anatomic structures, and

20

PATHOLOGY

21

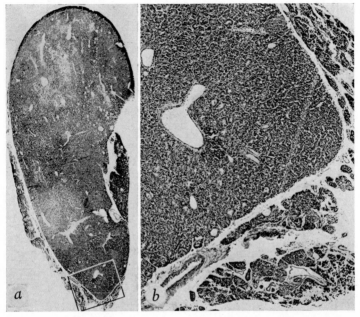

Fig. 2. Chief-cell adenoma with remnant of parathyroid gland. The fat-containing stroma is virtually absent within the adenoma. In *b* the rectangle at the bottom of *a* is shown at a higher magnification (*a*, x8; *b*, x50).

consequently are flattened, elongated or otherwise distorted. When the parent gland is situated in loose areolar tissue, the adenoma is ovoid or globular. Larger adenomas tend to be displaced into regions occupied by areolar tissue. They retain their ovoid shape and show only surface molding. There is a definite vascular pedicle which is more apparent in the case of larger, displaced tumors than in that of small adenomas adherent to the capsule of the thyroid. The capsule of the adenoma is thin and delicate but very definite. There is no attachment to surrounding structures except at the pedicle, unless inflammatory adhesions have developed as a consequence of degenerative changes within the adenoma. Such degenerative changes as cysts and calcification are common, particularly in larger tumors.

The most characteristic gross feature of a parathyroid adenoma is its yellowish brown or chocolate brown color. The color is definitely browner than that of the thyroid and is far darker than the color of lymph nodes or of the thymus. The distinctive color is readily obscured by hemorrhage into the adenoma or into the surrounding tissues. The characteristic color may be lost if extensive degenerative changes, particularly calcification, have occurred within the adenoma. Because of the loss of the brown color, calcified adenomas may be indistinguishable grossly from calcified adenomas of the thyroid, from lymph nodes or from other tissues.

On microscopic examination, adenomatous tissue is easily distinguished from normal parathyroid tissue by the virtual absence of fat in the former (Fig. 2). Roughly half of the bulk of a normal parathyroid of an adult is fat-containing stroma. The parenchyma is everywhere divided into masses and cords of cells by the fat-containing stroma, giving the section an over-all lacelike appearance. The parenchyma of an adenoma, in marked contrast, is made up of a solid mass as of cells. The stroma is not prominent, contains practically no fat and seems just sufficient to surround relatively large vessels. The absence of fat accounts for the fact that adenomatous tissue has a deeper brown color than that of a normal parathyroid, the color of the parenchyma of which is diluted by that of the yellow adipose tissue.

The parenchymal cells of a parathyroid adenoma differ little from those of a normal parathyroid of an adult. There is, however, more pleomorphism, giant nuclei are commoner, as are hyperchromatism and mitoses. The adenomatous tissue, while varying somewhat from area to area,

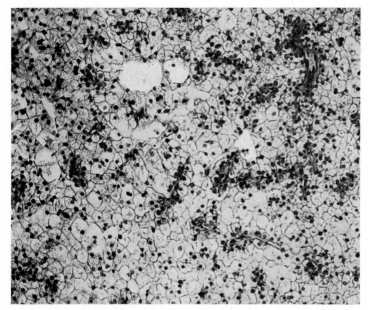

Fig. 3. Parathyroid adenoma, wasserhelle-cell type. The cells are smaller and less uniform than the cells of wasserhelle-cell hyperplasia. Many chief cells are present (x150).

tends to be of one cell type so that histologic classification of adenomas is possible. The type most commonly found is the chief-cell adenoma which, along with transitional chief-cell adenomas, accounts for more than 90 per cent of cases (Fig. 2). Transitional wasserhelle-cell adenomas (Fig. 3) and transitional oxyphil-cell adenomas (Fig. 4), while less common, are not unusual. In neither type are chief cells ever entirely absent. Castleman and Mallory[31] (1935) stated that all adenomas contain chief cells and proposed this as further evidence that all types of cells of the parathyroid parenchyma are derived from the chief cell.

There is no correlation between the histologic character of the adenoma and the intensity of the hyperparathy-

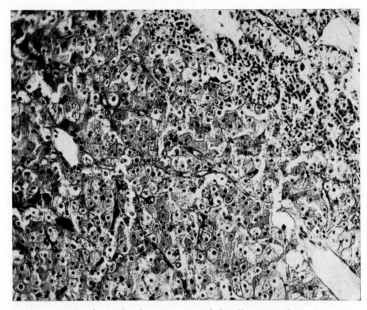

FIG. 4. Parathyroid adenoma, oxyphil-cell type. There are many chief cells in the upper right hand corner of the section. The transition between the oxyphils and the chief cells is abrupt (x150).

roidism. Oxyphil cells probably do not produce hormone,[31] so that the hyperparathyroidism caused by adenomas made up almost wholly of oxyphil cells results from the function of the other types of cells in the adenomas. Wasserhelle-cell adenomas present a special problem to the tissue pathologist because of the close resemblance of such adenomatous cells to those of wasserhelle hyperplasia. The adenomatous cells are usually smaller and exhibit more variation in type and size than the cells of the hyperplastic parathyroids, but the differences are relative at best (Fig. 3).

MULTIPLE ADENOMAS

Multiple adenomas and secondary hyperplasia of the parathyroid glands may be virtually indistinguishable on

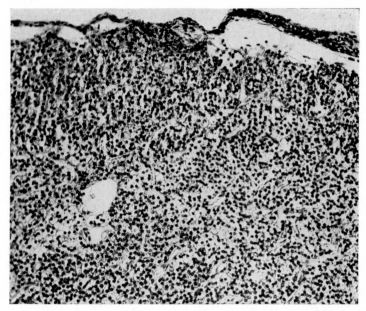

Fig. 5. Secondary hyperplasia. The great majority of cells are of the transitional wasserhelle type. Stromal fat is virtually absent (x150).

microscopic examination. Stromal fat, virtually absent in adenomatous tissue, may be greatly reduced in secondary hyperplasia. There are no essential differences in the parenchymal cells in the two lesions although the predominant cell in secondary hyperplasia tends to be the transitional wasserhelle cell[49] (Fig. 5). Furthermore, secondary hyperplasia is to be expected in cases of renal insufficiency,[32] and renal insufficiency is commonly observed in hyperparathyroidism. The confusion between the two lesions is understandable, as is the skepticism concerning the existence of multiple adenomas in cases of hyperparathyroidism. Norris (1947), for example, found reports of 20 cases of multiple adenomas among 322 cases of hyperfunctioning adenomas. All but two of the cases were from the older literature and had been reported before the present development of the knowledge of parathyroid pathology. Norris concluded that there was little evidence for the existence of multiple adenomas.

In the Mayo Clinic series of 112 cases, there have been 10 cases of multiple adenomas. In none of the 10 could the multiple tumors be accounted for reasonably on the basis of secondary hyperplasia due to renal insufficiency. In two cases, in both of which treatment was done before the occurrence of multiple adenomas had been widely recognized, the values for calcium and phosphorus in the serum were unaffected by the removal of one adenoma. This would seem conclusive evidence for the existence of at least one other adenoma. In another case a single adenoma had been removed elsewhere without influencing the hypercalcemia. The second adenoma was removed at the clinic with subsequent cure. In four cases, two adenomas were removed, cure resulting in each case. In two cases three adenomas were removed, and in the last case three adenomas were removed and the fourth was resected subtotally. In each of the three cases the patient was cured. Such cases demonstrate that multiple adenomas occur and that the removal of one of the adenomas does not cure the patient.

There are no fundamental differences, microscopic or gross, between single and multiple adenomas. The usual parathyroid tumor is a true solitary adenoma. Less commonly, the single tumor is apparently made up of multiple nodules, comparable to multiple nodular goiter. When tumors involve more than one gland they are quite likely to be of the multiple adenomatous type rather than of the single adenomatous type. In the multiple adenomatous tumors there is often an abrupt transition in type of cell from nodule to nodule so that nodules of wasserhelle cells may be contiguous to a nodule composed of chief cells. Multiple adenomatosis of a single parathyroid should suggest the possibility of similar involvement of other parathyroids. The finding of a true single adenoma in one parathyroid, unfortunately, however, does not preclude another adenoma in another gland.

PRIMARY HYPERPLASIA

Primary or wasserhelle hyperplasia was first described by Albright, Bloomberg, Castleman and Churchill in 1934. Rogers and Keating (1947) found reports of 22 cases in the literature and added four more from the Mayo Clinic. Primary hyperplasia is to be expected in somewhat less than 10 per cent of cases of hyperparathyroidism (eight of 89 cases in the Massachusetts General Hospital series; nine of 112 cases in the Mayo Clinic series). The hyperparathyroidism resulting from primary hyperplasia is indistinguishable from that caused by an adenoma.

All parathyroid tissue is involved. The different glands, however, may not be enlarged to the same extent. Rarely, one or more than one gland may be little if any enlarged; the hyperplastic cells merely replace the stromal fat without causing a gross increase in the size of the gland. The total weight of resected tissue in the clinic series has varied from 1.4 gm. to 52.5 gm. Grossly, the chocolate brown color is even more striking than that of adenomas. The parathyroid glands may be so enlarged that the glands on one side become fused. Masses of hyperplastic tissue may be lobulated, and cysts, areas of calcification and pseudopods are common.

Microscopically, the only cell seen is the water-clear or wasserhelle cell (Fig. 6). The cells are sharply demarcated and average about 20 microns in diameter. The nucleus is

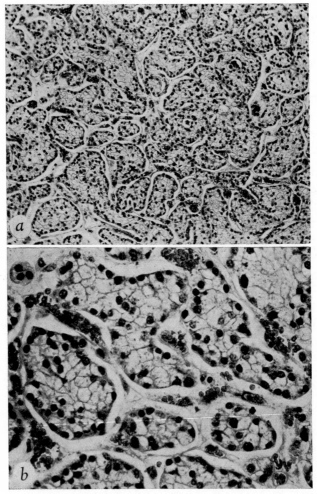

Fig. 6. Primary or wasserhelle-cell hyperplasia. The uniform cellu-
lar pattern and pseudoglandular arrangement of the cells are typical.
The cells are larger, more uniform and more regularly distributed
than the cells of a wasserhelle-cell adenoma (*a*, x120; *b*, x350).

approximately the size of the nucleus of a chief cell and stands out clearly from the remainder of the cell, which appears empty. The nucleus is often in the end of the tall cell toward the stroma, giving the appearance of a "branch of berries" (Castleman and Mallory). The appearance of the cells has been compared to that of the cells of clear-cell carcinomas of the kidney. There is some variation in the size of the cells, but on the whole, the microscopic appearance is essentially the same throughout the tissue.[13] The stroma, composed of thin fibrous tissue, is increased in amount and surrounds varying-sized groups of cells. Together with the characteristic basilar orientation of the nuclei, this produces a pseudoglandular or acinar effect. The typical appearance is best shown in paraffin sections. However, if fresh tissue is fixed for two or three minutes in boiling formalin before frozen sections are made, the architecture of the cells is well preserved and the wasserhelle cells are easily recognized.

As previously mentioned, adenomas may be almost entirely made up of wasserhelle cells. It is imperative to distinguish at the time of operation between such an adenoma and wasserhelle hyperplasia. In the majority of cases of primary hyperplasia this offers little difficulty because of the obvious enlargement of all glands. In cases in which one gland only is apparently involved, biopsy of specimens taken from other glands will aid materially in differentiating conditions with certainty.

CARCINOMA

Hyperfunctioning carcinomas of parathyroid origin which infiltrate, recur and metastasize are fortunately rare. Such lesions account for perhaps 1 per cent of cases of hyperparathyroidism (one case in 89, Massachusetts General Hospital series; one case in 112, Mayo Clinic

series). The case of Meyer, Rosi and Ragins, first reported
in 1939, dispelled all skepticism concerning the existence
of such lesions. At least 12 other cases have been reported
since in which a hyperfunctioning malignant tumor infiltrated locally or metastasized.[25] Extensive local recurrence has been reported more often than distant metastasis. In cases in which metastatic growths have occurred,
cervical and mediastinal nodes have been involved most
frequently, pulmonary metastatic growths are known to
have developed in three cases, and in one case a kidney
was involved metastatically. By the time metastatic
growths have developed or the lesion has infiltrated sur-

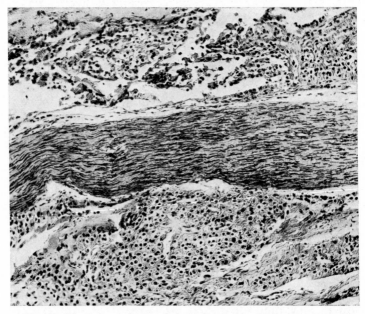

Fig. 7. Carcinoma of parathyroid origin showing neural involvement. The cytologic architecture is not strikingly different from
that of many adenomas which have neither metastasized nor re-
curred (x120).

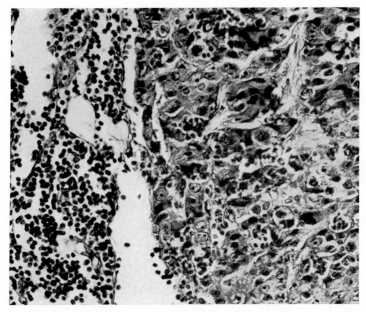

FIG. 8. Metastatic parathyroid carcinoma in lymph node (x285).

rounding structures, it has probably become incurable. The case of Gentile, Skinner and Ashburn (1941) possibly is an exception, but the serum calcium was elevated, the serum phosphorus was depressed and the skeleton had not recalcified completely five years after the first operation. Patients may survive for prolonged periods but die eventually, usually of renal insufficiency or hypertension due to recurrent or persistent hyperparathyroidism. In the single case in the Mayo Clinic series, death occurred eight years after the onset of the osseous disease and six years after the first operation. The lesion responds little, if at all, to external irradiation.

On microscopic examination, the cytologic architecture is not markedly different from that of the usual adenoma (Figs. 7 and 8). Indeed, this similarity has given rise to a controversy which is as yet unsettled. Alexander and his colleagues (1944), on purely cytologic evidence, considered the tumors in 12 of the first 14 cases of hyperparathyroidism in the Mayo Clinic series to be carcinomas of low grade. Sufficient time has elapsed, and an adequate number of cases have been observed, to demonstrate that the usual adenoma neither recurs nor metastasizes. However, the histopathologic characteristics of certain adenomas have proved very similar to those of carcinomas which have metastasized. The question is of less practical importance at present than formerly, since the practice of resecting adenomas subtotally has been largely abandoned.

Chapter V

CLINICAL ASPECTS

THE SYMPTOMS of hyperparathyroidism are of three types: those caused by the hypercalcemia, those pertaining to the urinary tract and those of the osseous complications.[73] Four variations of the disease, consequently, may be seen clinically: (1) hyperparathyroidism with complications involving the urinary tract; (2) hyperparathyroidism with osseous complications; (3) hyperparathyroidism with both osseous and renal complications; and (4) hyperparathyroidism with neither osseous nor renal complications. The first type is by far the commonest, while the "classic type" of the older literature—that is, generalized osteitis fibrosa—is less common (Table II). By the time generalized osteitis fibrosa has developed, urinary complications are frequently found, although changes in the urinary tract may be absent even with advanced osseous disease.

TABLE II. CLINICAL MANIFESTATIONS IN 112 PROVED CASES OF HYPERPARATHYROIDISM*

Generalized osteitis fibrosa	16†
Generalized osteitis fibrosa and renal involvement	16
Renal involvement (urinary lithiasis, calcinosis or both)	73
Neither renal nor osseous involvement	7

Polyendocrine adenomas	3
Osteoporosis	2
Convulsive disorder	1
Tumor found at thyroidectomy	1

Total	112

* Osseous disease evident roentgenographically as generalized osteitis fibrosa in 30 per cent of cases, renal involvement in 80 per cent of cases.
† Includes one case of polyendocrine adenoma.

In the absence of both osseous and renal complications the diagnosis is usually made almost by accident in that calcium determination has been ordered with some other condition in mind. The demonstration of hypercalcemia has then suggested the possibility of hyperparathyroidism. In the Mayo Clinic series, the patients in whom the diagnosis has been made in the absence of complications have usually had convulsions.[96] The serum calcium determinations were ordered originally with the convulsions of tetany in mind.

AGE

Hyperparathyroidism may occur at any age from childhood on. The diagnosis in children is more difficult than in adults, essentially because of the labile metabolism of calcium and phosphorus during growth. Neither the case reported by Landon (1932) of hyperparathyroidism involving a 2½-year-old child, nor the case of Anspach and Clifton (1939) involving an infant of 11 months was proved. The correct diagnosis in Duken's case (1928) involving a child of seven years proved at necropsy to be sarcomatosis. Anspach and Clifton, however, found reports of 11 other cases in the literature involving children. The youngest patient in the Mayo Clinic series was 14 years of age at the time the diagnosis was made. Her symptoms probably started at about 12 years of age. The disease is commoner after 20 years of age, and reaches a peak in the sixth decade (Fig. 9). The ages given are those at the time the diagnosis was established.

SEX

The sexes are affected equally. In the Mayo Clinic series there are 57 men and 55 women. This is at variance with the usual statement in the literature that the condition occurs more frequently in women than in men. General-

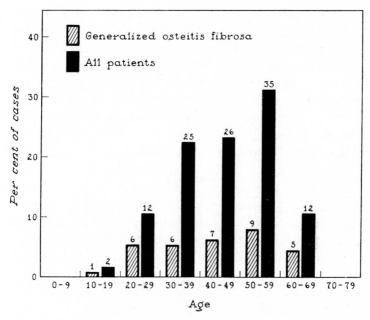

FIG. 9. Ages of patients at time of treatment. The numbers above columns are the number of patients at the indicated age. Hyperparathyroidism is unusual before 20 years of age, and usually occurs between the ages of 30 and 60 years.

ized osteitis fibrosa does occur more often in women than in men, the ratio being approximately two to one. However, complications involving the urinary tract develop more frequently in men than in women, the sex ratio being almost reversed. Since renal complications are commoner than generalized osteitis fibrosa, the disease probably will be found, as more cases are accumulated, to occur more frequently in men than in women.

DURATION OF SYMPTOMS

Data concerning duration of symptoms are fundamentally unsatisfactory in hyperparathyroidism as in most other chronic diseases. In the Mayo Clinic series, the duration of symptoms varied from 10 days to 32 years. Among patients with generalized osteitis fibrosa the average was 4.5 years; the shortest duration was just less than one year and the longest more than 10 years. Among patients with renal complications, the diagnosis was established in one case 10 days after the first renal colic. At the opposite extreme, one patient had had recurrent renal colics for 27 years and another for 32 years before the diagnosis was made. Since in all cases, at least before extensive renal damage has been produced, there is a continuously increased excretion of calcium and phosphorus in the urine, renal stones and renal calcinosis may develop at any time. Conversely, demineralization of the skeleton requires an interval of time for its development.

SYMPTOMS DUE TO HYPERCALCEMIA

The increased concentration of ionic calcium in the serum is associated with a decrease in neuromuscular excitability to both mechanical and electrical stimuli. This results in hypotonia involving all muscles. The clinical manifestations of this in skeletal muscles are weakness, easy fatigue and hypermobility of the joints, which may be sufficiently marked to produce disturbances in gait. In smooth muscle, the hypotonicity is responsible for distention, constipation and anorexia. Nausea and vomiting, usually in attacks, are not uncommon. The impaired function of the bowel probably accounts for the moderate loss of weight which is usually observed. The changes in cardiac muscle are demonstrable electrocardiographically in a shortening of the Q-T interval (shortened ventricular systole) which, however, rarely exceeds normal limits.

The symptoms are proportional to the degree of the hypercalcemia. In cases in which the calcium is little elevated, the symptoms are correspondingly mild and may not even be recognized by the patient. In cases in which the hypercalcemia is marked, the symptoms are more definite. However, in such cases they are usually overshadowed by the more painful symptoms caused by urinary or skeletal complications which are likely to have developed. The symptoms of hypercalcemia resemble in general those of common, purely functional, conditions and serve usually to confuse rather than to help one in making the diagnosis.[74] The true importance of the symptoms often becomes evident only when they are appraised in retrospect after correction of the hypercalcemia. The disappearance of the chronic fatigue and gaseous indigestion, the improvement in muscular tone and strength, and the gain of weight are often striking.

SYMPTOMS ASSOCIATED WITH THE URINARY TRACT

The urinary symptoms of hyperparathyroidism are polyuria and polydypsia, those of urinary calculi, and those produced by deposits of calcium in the tubules of the kidneys (nephrocalcinosis[6]) (Fig. 10).

Polyuria and polydypsia result from the primary action of the parathyroid hormone, which has a definite diuretic effect. In addition to increasing the excretion of calcium and phosphorus in the urine, the hormone causes an increased loss of water, chlorides and fixed base.[103] The hormone has been used clinically as a diuretic agent. In cases of hyperparathyroidism in which renal function is impaired, the tubular damage probably also contributes to the increased formation of urine. The polyuria and polydypsia may be sufficiently marked to suggest diabetes insipidus. In the usual case of mild hyperparathyroidism, however, the amount of urine may not be sufficiently large

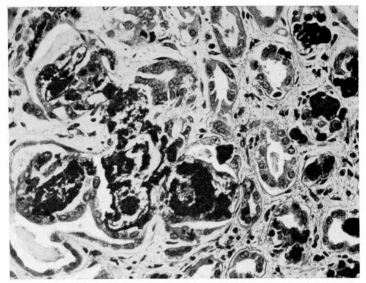

Fig. 10. Nephrocalcinosis in acute hyperparathyroidism. Patient
died of renal insufficiency (x235).

to attract the patient's attention. In such cases, the oliguria
which develops promptly after the removal of the hyperfunctioning tissue is much more striking. The postoperative development of oliguria is the first clinical evidence
that the hyperparathyroidism has been corrected. If the
volume of urine does not decrease immediately after removal of a parathyroid adenoma, there is strong presumptive evidence that not all hyperfunctioning tissue has been
removed. In the usual case, in which the value for calcium
in the serum is perhaps 12 to 13 mg. per 100 cc., the intravenous administration of 2 liters of fluid during the
first 12 hours after operation is followed by the excretion of
as little as 500 to 600 cc. of urine.

The formation of calculi is the commonest complication
of hyperparathyroidism. The stones presumably result
from the increased excretion of calcium and phosphorus

in the urine, so that calcium phosphate and calcium oxalate stones would be expected. In alkaline urines, stones of ammonium-magnesium phosphate also form. The pure character of the stones is lost after the development of infection and stasis. Stag-horn calculi are unusual but occasionally develop. The passage of sand and gravel is common. As previously mentioned, stones may develop at any time during the course of the disease.[2] Recurrent lithiasis is to be expected, since stones continue to form as long as the hypercalciuria persists, and should suggest hyperparathyroidism more strongly than the passage of a single stone. Beard and Goodyear (1950) have recently re-emphasized the fact that hyperparathyroidism should be considered in all cases of renal lithiasis and not only in cases of recurrent or multiple lithiasis. In two thirds of their cases a single stone only had formed.

The precipitation of calcium and phosphorus to form stones is dependent, at least in part, on their concentration in the urine. If the urine is sufficiently dilute, precipitation is unusual. Freeman (1949), studying stone formation in recumbent patients, found that urinary stones rarely formed when the concentration of calcium in the urine was kept below 150 mg. per liter. Dilution of urine may account for the fact that stones fail to form, or form rarely, in an occasional case of hyperparathyroidism. The dilute urine of renal insufficiency may also explain the tendency for patients with calcinosis not to form stones.

Renal calcinosis, or the deposition of calcium in the tubules of the kidney, is probably the most serious complication of hyperparathyroidism. Why calcinosis occurs in some cases and lithiasis in others is not known, nor is it known why patients may have hyperparathyroidism with urinary lithiasis for years and yet not develop calcinosis. Calcinosis, evident roentgenologically, is less common than lithiasis and is more likely to develop in cases in which the serum calcium is high than in cases in which it is low.

The amount of calcium in the kidneys does not decrease, as judged roentgenographically, after cure of the hyperparathyroidism. Renal calcinosis is invariably associated with some impairment of renal function. In such cases, renal function may improve somewhat after cure of the hyperparathyroidism. In most cases, however, the improvement is slight or does not occur. It is becoming increasingly evident from follow-up studies that the impairment of renal function may be progressive in spite of the fact that the hyperparathyroidism has been cured. Rienhoff (1949) found that nine of 25 patients cured of hyperparathyroidism had died between three and 11 years after operation. Death in all cases resulted from hypertension or renal insufficiency. Hellstrom (1950) reviewed the late results after treatment in 21 cases. He concluded that the ultimate outcome of the case was dependent on the renal damage at the time of operation. The slow progressive decrease of renal function ultimately resulting in the death of a patient cured of hyperparathyroidism is well illustrated by the following case from the Mayo Clinic series.

REPORT OF A CASE

The patient was a woman aged 21 years who had developed symptoms associated with generalized osteitis fibrosa five or six years before admission. In addition to advanced osseous changes, moderate renal calcinosis was found roentgenographically. The calcium averaged 15.8 mg. and the phosphorus 2.9 mg. per 100 cc. of serum. The value for alkaline phosphatase was 19.1 Bodansky units. A parathyroid adenoma which weighed 6 gm. was removed in June, 1941. The hyperparathyroidism re-

mained cured. The patient was seen at the clinic from
time to time during the succeeding seven years. The value
for urea in the blood was 50 mg. per 100 cc. at the time
of the operation. Four years later the value had risen to
80, and one year later was 140 mg. per 100 cc. The blood
pressure was 126 mm. of mercury systolic and 84 diastolic
at the time the diagnosis of hyperparathyroidism was established. Four years later the values were 152 and 94,
a year later 170 and 90. Fairly marked polyuria had meanwhile developed. The patient died elsewhere eight and
a half years after the operation, at the age of 30 years,
from renal insufficiency.

There seems little doubt that renal insufficiency due to
calcinosis, at least beyond a certain point, is progressive
in spite of any treatment. If death is to be prevented,
treatment of the hyperparathyroidism must be carried out
before the stage of progressive renal insufficiency has been
reached.

SYMPTOMS DUE TO OSSEOUS COMPLICATIONS

The skeletal changes of hyperparathyroidism are often
entirely absent. As discussed previously, there are no demonstrable skeletal changes so long as the intake of calcium is equal to the loss of calcium. If the calcium balance
becomes negative, either because of diminished intake or
absorption, or because of increased loss of calcium, the
deficit is made up by absorption from the skeleton. A large
intake of calcium, as is the case with milk drinkers,[3] may
protect the skeleton in even fairly severe hyperparathyroidism, whereas if the diet is low in calcium, less marked
degrees of hypercalciuria will be associated with demineralization. Skeletal changes are more likely to develop
in severe cases since a positive calcium balance is less
likely to be maintained than in less severe cases. It fol-

lows that the absence of osseous lesions has no bearing on diagnosis.

Since hyperparathyroidism is a systemic disease the osseous changes, when present, must involve the entire skeleton. The fundamental change is demineralization, which affects all bones. Changes secondary to the demineralization may be localized. They are often far more striking than the generalized demineralization and may give the erroneous impression that the osseous changes are localized. The secondary changes are deformities, cysts, tumors, changes in the internal architecture of bone and fractures. They are most obvious in bones subject to weight bearing such as the bones of the legs and pelvis and the vertebrae.

The demineralized skeleton is painful and tender; the tenderness is quite marked and of diagnostic importance. Early in the course of the skeletal disease the discomfort is often diagnosed erroneously as arthritis or neuritis. As the disease progresses the tenderness of the bones should make such an impression untenable. Fractures, which often occur at the site of a cyst or tumor, are associated with the usual findings and the usual amount of pain. They heal normally, unless repair is prevented by the cyst or tumor. The deformities may involve any bone but are likely to be most manifest in the bones of the legs and the vertebrae. The nucleus pulposus pushes deeply into the body of the softened vertebrae so that the body may appear as a biconcave disk. These changes, together with crushing of vertebrae, which is common, may lead to marked loss of height. In advanced cases the neck seems to be lost in the chest. Tumors and cysts are particularly common in the jaw, pelvis and the ends of the long bones. The cortex is often expanded over the larger cysts. In advanced cases, there is a marked increase of fibrous tissue which encroaches on the marrow space and leads to secondary anemia.

Roentgenologic Findings: The roentgenologic findings vary from none to those of advanced generalized osteitis fibrosa. In the Mayo Clinic series, less than 30 per cent of cases had generalized osteitis fibrosa recognizable as such by the roentgenologist. In another 20 to 30 per cent of cases some demineralization of the skeleton was thought to have been apparent roentgenographically, and in the remaining cases, roughly one half of the group, no change in the skeleton was reported in the records. It is possible that the proportion of cases with roentgenographically recognizable changes could have been increased by more extended study of the skeleton. That such extensive studies were not thought necessary is an indication of the changed emphasis in diagnosis from roentgenologic to laboratory studies.

While the skeletal involvement is generalized in those cases in which there is skeletal disease, the generalized involvement may not be evident roentgenographically.[87] With minimal osseous disease much of the skeleton may appear normal. In such cases, certain parts of the skeleton show the changes of hyperparathyroidism more definitely roentgenographically than others. These are the hands, the periodontal osseous tissue and the calvarium. These regions should be included in any roentgenographic survey of the skeleton for hyperparathyroidism.

According to Pugh[87] (1951) the most important and dependable roentgenographic evidence of hyperparathyroidism is subperiosteal resorption of bone. It is seen most frequently along the margins of the middle phalanges of the fingers. All phalanges are usually involved, but in minimal cases it shows best in the middle phalanges. The characteristic change is not merely decalcification of the cortex but a peculiar lacelike decalcification of the cortical bone just beneath the periosteum (Fig. 11). It is seen in no other condition except renal rickets, in which it is a manifesta-

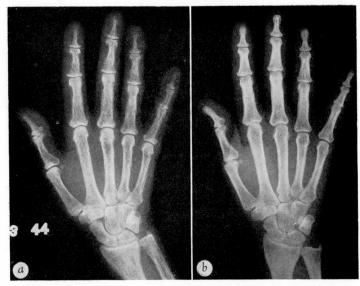

FIG. 11. *a*. Generalized osteitis fibrosa. In addition to generalized demineralization, the characteristic lacelike subcortical resorption of the phalanges is well illustrated. There is also resorption of the terminal phalanges and gross derangement of the internal architecture of the bones. *b*. Thirteen months after cure of hyperparathyroidism. Bones of normal density. Internal architecture almost normal. Some evidence of healed generalized osteitis fibrosa in middle and proximal phalanges.

tion of secondary hyperparathyroidism. In addition the roentgenograms of the hands show demineralization and deranged internal architecture and may show resorption of the terminal tufts of the distal phalanges and subperiosteal cysts.

The subperiosteal resorption appears next best in the osseous tissue around the teeth. The periodontal membrane, which surrounds the root or roots of each tooth, appears black on dental roentgenograms. This is a specialized periosteum covering a layer of cortical bone which forms the socket of the tooth. This layer of bone is called

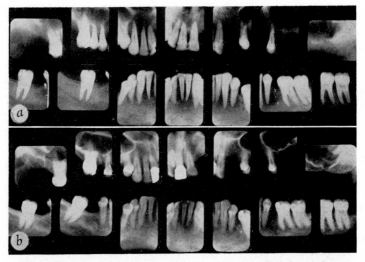

Fig. 12. Dental roentgenograms. *a*. Absence of lamina dura in generalized osteitis fibrosa. *b*. Its regeneration after cure of the hyperparathyroidism.

the lamina dura and appears roentgenographically as a well-defined white line. Subperiosteal absorption causes the lamina dura to disappear (Fig. 12). Absence of the lamina dura is a less reliable sign of hyperparathyroidism than subperiosteal resorption in the phalanges, since the lamina dura may not be evident roentgenographically in many other conditions. Diagnosis from dental roentgenograms is more accurate if the surrounding osseous tissue is considered in addition to the lamina dura. The surrounding trabecular structure is lost and anatomic landmarks such as the inferior dental canal, the mental foramen and the floor of the antrum are indistinct. Keating (1947) has pointed out that the teeth, which do not decalcify, provide an excellent index to the degree of decalcification of the surrounding bone.

The diagnostic importance of the appearance of the cal-

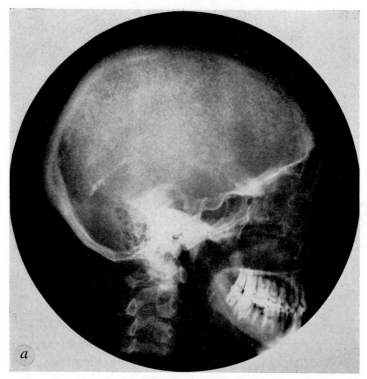

Fig. 13. Changes in the skull in generalized osteitis fibrosa. *a.* "Ground-glass" demineralization. *b.* Remineralization three years after cure of hyperparathyroidism. Architecture not normal, evidence of healed generalized osteitis fibrosa.

varium was emphasized by Camp and Ochsner (1931) more than twenty years ago. The texture of the bone of the calvarium is quite distinctive and, in advanced cases, almost diagnostic (Fig. 13). In typical cases, there is a characteristic granular or miliary decalcification to which the term "ground-glass appearance" has been applied. The inner and outer tables, as well as the vascular markings, become indistinct. There may be associated cysts which

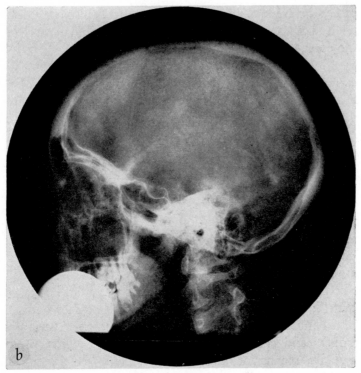

See legend on opposite page.

further suggest the diagnosis. Occasionally, in far-advanced cases, the skull may be thickened and resemble somewhat that of Paget's disease.

In cases in which there is obvious abnormality of bone, the roentgenologic diagnosis is not particularly difficult. In addition to the changes previously discussed, the whole skeleton is demineralized, trabeculae appear indistinct and fuzzy, and the normal trabecular structure is grossly deranged. The cortex of the long bones is thinned, and the bones appear without much trabecular structure. In other cases, the trabeculae, though fuzzy and not sharply out-lined, appear coarse and prominent. Cystlike lesions of the cortex are common and are most suggestive of hyper-parathyroidism. Pathologic fractures are also common and contribute to the gross deformities of the skeleton. Calci-fication of the soft tissue is usually not apparent roentgeno-graphically except for calcification of the kidneys in cases in which renal calcinosis has developed. Intra-articular and periarticular deposits of calcium may be found rarely. They are more characteristic of other conditions than of hyperparathyroidism.

Cured generalized osteitis fibrosa is also recognizable roentgenographically. The true cysts do not recalcify, but the cystlike areas caused by osteoblastomas become densely calcified. The deformities remain, but the internal architecture of the bone gradually reverts toward normal. The organic matrix has usually been so altered, however, that the texture of the bone never quite becomes normal. The lamina dura reappears. The process requires many months and can be followed both roentgenographically and by means of alkaline phosphatase levels, which remain elevated until the skeletal repair has been com-pleted.

ACUTE HYPERPARATHYROIDISM

Acute hyperparathyroidism or acute parathyroid poison-ing was first produced experimentally by Collip, Clark and Scott (1925). They found that massive doses of parathyroid extract caused anuria and death within a few days. The blood of the experimental animals became so inspissated that samples for analysis were difficult to take. Shelling, Kajdi and Guth (1938) demonstrated that the inspissation of the blood resulted from the marked diuresis produced by the hormone. They were able to prevent death by replacing the lost fluid and electrolytes. Tweedy, Templeton and McJunkin (1936) found that nephrectomy protected dogs from the effects of overdosage with parathyroid extract. It is probable that the inspissation of the blood resulting from the diuretic effect of the hormone interferes with renal function to the point that both calcium and phosphorus are retained. At some critical level precipitation occurs in the tissues. The precipitation of calcium in the tubules of the kidneys causes irreversible renal damage which, if extensive enough, causes death. Up to a point the condition is reversible, as demonstrated by Shelling and his colleagues (1938). Probably the first case in man was reported by Dawson and Struthers (1923) and other cases have been since reported by Hanes (1939), by Oliver (1939), and by Smith and Cooke (1940). Rogers (1946) reported data on two other cases proved at necropsy and reviewed the literature to that time.

The condition is far more important clinically than the few reported cases would suggest. In any case of hyperparathyroidism, particularly in cases in which the serum calcium is unusually high and associated with some impairment of renal function, which is not unusual, dehydration can initiate the cycle leading to renal failure and death. In one of the Mayo Clinic cases, reported by Rogers (1946), for example, the upset of fluid balance after gastric resection was sufficient to bring about acute renal calcinosis which resulted in the death of the patient from renal insufficiency. The existence of the hyperparathyroidism in this case was not suspected before the necropsy was performed.

In spite of the fact that many surgical procedures, particularly operations on the urinary tract, have been carried out successfully in cases of hyperparathyroidism, it would seem much safer to postpone such operations until after the hyperparathyroidism has been corrected. The chance of

precipitating acute hyperparathyroidism by a surgical procedure on the urinary tract is still another reason why
hyperparathyroidism should be excluded before any operation for renal lithiasis is undertaken. The same changes
can be initiated by injudicious treatment with calcium,
milk or vitamin D, which are all too readily prescribed to
treat the obviously demineralized skeleton of generalized
osteitis fibrosa. Any agent which could increase the level
of calcium or phosphorus is contraindicated in hyperparathyroidism. The logical treatment, prior to parathyroid
surgery, would be directed toward limiting the intake of
calcium and phosphorus, and promoting their excretion by
means of a large intake of fluids.

PEPTIC ULCER AND HYPERPARATHYROIDISM

The association of peptic ulcer and hyperparathyroidism
was pointed out first by Rogers (1946) and by Rogers,
Keating, Morlock and Barker (1947). Similar cases have
been since reported by others.[22, 99] The three cases reported
by Rogers and his colleagues led to a review of all cases of
hyperparathyroidism in the Mayo Clinic series by Haynes
(1950). He found that 24 per cent of patients with proved
hyperparathyroidism had at the time of examination, or
had had in the past, objective evidence of peptic ulcer or
had had operations on the stomach, presumably because
of ulcer. An additional 15 to 20 per cent of patients had
had some ulcer-like symptoms but an ulcer had never been
proved. The ulcers were duodenal rather than gastric in
the great majority of proved cases, although there were a
few gastric ulcers in the series. In several cases in the series, including two necropsy cases in which the hyperparathyroidism was not recognized before death, there were
peptic ulcers but no history of urinary lithiasis. It is tempt-
ing to propose that careful screening of patients with pep-

tic ulcer for hyperparathyroidism would yield cases of hyperparathyroidism which are not being recognized at present.

The explanation for the association is not clear. Rogers and his collaborators (1947) speculated as to whether prolonged treatment of the ulcer with calcium could in some way have led to the parathyroid hyperfunction. Several cases in the Mayo Clinic series suggest that ulcer treatment, either medical or surgical, is less satisfactory in patients who have hyperparathyroidism than treatment after the hyperparathyroidism has been cured. One patient, for example, had had moderately severe ulcer symptoms for three years before removal of a parathyroid adenoma. He has had no symptoms since the operation. In another case a jejunal ulcer, the crater of which was demonstrable roentgenologically, developed within six weeks after an adequate partial gastrectomy had been carried out elsewhere. On examination at the clinic, the patient was found to have hyperparathyroidism in addition to the jejunal ulcer. The pain associated with the ulcer had almost completely subsided and the ulcer crater had become smaller within two weeks after removal of a hyperfunctioning adenoma. The crater of the ulcer was not demonstrable elsewhere three months postoperatively. The patient had been on a careful ulcer program before and after the treatment of the hyperparathyroidism. Schneider and Robnett (1951) have recently reported another case in which response to treatment of the ulcer was poor until the hyperparathyroidism had been corrected, when the symptoms due to the ulcer regressed rapidly.

Schriffrin (1942) and others have demonstrated definite changes in the volume, acidity and pepsin activity in gastric secretions after injections of parathyroid extract. Such findings, coupled with the limited clinical observations, suggest that hyperparathyroidism may in some fashion predispose to peptic ulceration.

HYPERPARATHYROIDISM AND POLYENDOCRINE ADENOMAS*

Among the 112 cases in the Mayo Clinic series, there are four in which the hyperparathyroidism was associated with adenomas of other endocrine glands.[96] In all four cases there were hyperfunctioning tumors of the islet cells of the pancreas; in two of the four, in addition, there were pituitary tumors. One patient observed since 1949 had tumors of the parathyroid glands, the islet cells, the pituitary and one adrenal gland. The relationship is wholly inexplicable at this time. In one of the four cases generalized osteitis fibrosa had developed. In the other three, the outstanding symptom was convulsions due, in each case, to hypoglycemia. In the first of these three cases the hyperparathyroidism was recognized only because calcium determinations were carried out to exclude tetany as the cause of the convulsions. Subsequent cases were revealed through the screening of patients wih hypoglycemia by means of determinations of serum calcium. The cases are important with respect to the hyperparathyroidism in that the parathyroid adenomas are likely to be multiple and may even involve all four glands.

---

* Since this manuscript was completed the experience at the Mayo Clinic to date has been reported (Underdahl, L. O., Woolner, L. B. and Black, B. M.: Multiple Endocrine Adenomas: Report of Eight Cases in Which the Parathyroids, Pituitary and Pancreatic Islets Were Involved. *J. Clin. Endocrinol. & Metab.*, 13:20-47, Jan., 1953).

Chapter VI

DIAGNOSIS

EXCEPT in the relatively uncommon cases of full developed generalized osteitis fibrosa, the diagnosis of
hyperparathyroidism requires laboratory confirmation. The
condition, in the great majority of cases, cannot be recognized without laboratory aids. No single test is adequate
to establish the diagnosis; however, using a limited number
of different tests, the diagnosis can be made or excluded
with almost complete certainty. It would seem superfluous
to stress the fact that the tests must be accurate and consistent. Determinations of the level of calcium in the serum
are, however, notoriously inaccurate.[21] Unless such inaccu-
racies can be corrected, the diagnosis of hyperparathyroidism cannot even be seriously considered, much less acted
on. The following tests should be available: calcium in
serum and urine, phosphorus in serum, total proteins in
serum, blood urea or other tests by which renal function
may be evaluated, and alkaline phosphatase level in serum.

SERUM CALCIUM

In the Mayo Clinic series, calcium values have varied
from 10.6 to 17.8 mg. per 100 cc. of serum. Higher values
have been reported. Values of less than 11 mg. were found
in approximately 7 per cent of cases and values less than 11.5
mg. in 23 per cent of cases (Fig. 14). In our laboratories, the
upper limit of the normal range is closer to 10.5 than to 11
mg. per 100 cc. of serum, and any value greater than 10.5
mg. is regarded as being in the hypercalcemic range. Failure to appreciate that calcium values from 10.5 to 11.5 mg.
per 100 cc. of serum are compatible with the diagnosis of
hyperparathyroidism is a common error.

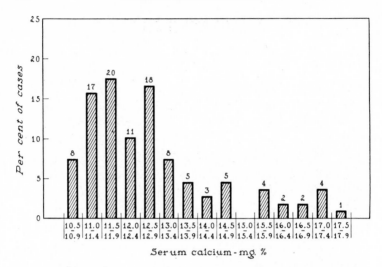

FIG. 14. Values for calcium in serum in 108 cases of hyperparathyroidism. The number above each column denotes the number
of cases in which the values for calcium were within the indicated
range.

The value for calcium in serum, as reported by the laboratory, is the total calcium in the serum. Only the ionic
calcium increases in hyperparathyroidism, whereas the
fraction bound to protein varies with the level of the serum
proteins. If the proteins are elevated, the serum calcium is
elevated and, conversely, if the protein is low the serum
calcium is low. It follows that in all cases of suspected
hyperparathyroidism the serum calcium must be considered in conjunction with the value for serum proteins.
Serum protein values sufficiently low to conceal the increased ionic calcium of hyperparathyroidism are most unusual. The reverse, in which the hypercalcemia is due to
an increase in the calcium proteinate fraction, is not unusual in conditions which may be confused with hyperparathyroidism. The two fractions can be determined di-

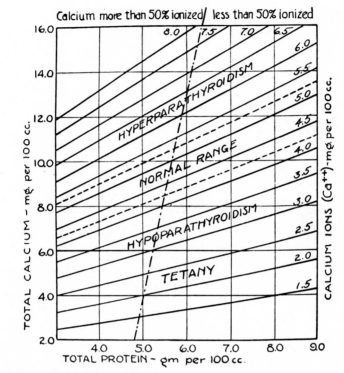

FIG. 15. Relationship of ionic calcium to total calcium and total proteins in serum. (From McLean, F. C. and Hastings, A. B.: *Am. J. M. Sc., 189*:601-613 (May) 1935, by permission of Lea & Febiger, publishers.)

rectly only with considerable difficulty. They may be calculated readily, however, from the nomogram of McLean and Hastings (1935) if the values for calcium and protein in the serum are known (Fig. 15). It is rarely necessary to secure the value for ionic calcium unless the serum proteins are definitely elevated. In such cases, serious diagnostic errors will be made unless the total serum calcium is considered in terms of the two fractions.

SERUM PHOSPHORUS (INORGANIC)

Except in cases of intoxication with vitamin D, the combination of hypercalcemia and hypophosphatemia is observed for practical purposes only in hyperparathyroidism. In the absence of renal insufficiency, values of less than 3.5 mg. per 100 cc. (1-2 mg. per 100 cc. higher in children) are found. With renal insufficiency phosphorus is retained so that normal values or even values well above the physiologic range may be found in cases of hyperparathyroidism. The weight given to the value for phosphorus in diagnosis depends, therefore, largely on the function of the kidneys. This may be assessed adequately for present purposes by the simple determination of the level of urea or nonprotein nitrogen. If the urea in the blood is elevated, the value for phosphorus may not be low. Conversely, if the urea is normal the value for phosphorus should be depressed. The value for phosphorus is of greatest importance diagnostically when the elevation of calcium is equivocal. In such cases, the hypophosphatemia may be more striking than the hypercalcemia. Such findings would rather be expected because of the primary action of the hormone on phosphorus rather than on calcium.

URINARY EXCRETION OF CALCIUM

Using the proper dose of parathyroid extract, the urinary excretion of calcium in normal persons may be doubled without altering appreciably the level of calcium in the serum.[11] Particularly in cases of mild hyperparathyroidism this marked effect on the excretion of calcium may provide the additional evidence necessary to establish the diagnosis. The test is carried out by placing the patient for three days on the diet described by Bauer and Aub (1927). All urine is collected and the amount of calcium in each

24-hour sample is determined. The values are averaged. The daily diet contains 125 mg. of calcium. The normal urinary excretion is less than 100 mg. per day. Values from 125 to 200 mg. per day are highly suspicious and values greater than 200 mg. per day are definitely abnormal.

The findings must be interpreted with much caution and only in conjunction with other clinical and laboratory data. Hypercalciuria occurs in any condition characterized by rapid demineralization of the skeleton, in renal acidosis, in idiopathic hypercalciuria and in other conditions. Idiopathic hypercalciuria is characterized by an abnormally high urinary excretion of calcium at a normal level of calcium in the serum. It is apparently a common finding in cases of urinary lithiasis. Flocks (1940) found an abnormally high excretion of calcium in the urine in two thirds of a group of patients with calcium nephrolithiasis, and in all cases in the group in which the stones were recurrent or were increasing rapidly in size. Hyperparathyroidism was excluded in all cases.

The Sulkowitch test[17] is not a substitute for calcium balance studies, nor is it a particularly effective screening test for hyperparathyroidism. The test is a crudely quantitative bedside method for determining the concentration of calcium in the urine. The results are affected by the concentration of the urine, by renal disease, by diet, by age and probably by other factors as well. A heavy precipitate of calcium in the urine signifies little from the standpoint of the diagnosis of hyperparathyroidism. A persistently low excretion in concentrated urine is, however, presumptive evidence against the diagnosis of hyperparathyroidism. It should be recalled that the urinary excretion of calcium may be decreased in renal insufficiency.

ALKALINE PHOSPHATASE

The value for alkaline phosphatase in the serum in the absence of hepatic disease or obstructive jaundice is a measure of osteoblastic activity. In hyperparathyroidism it is elevated in proportion to the extent of the osseous disease, and bears no other relation to the intensity of the hyperparathyroidism. The normal value in adults is 4.5 Bodansky units; in children values as high as 10 may be found. With extensive osseous changes values of 20 units or more may be observed. The values remain elevated after cure of the hyperparathyroidism and return only slowly to normal as the skeleton becomes remineralized. Pugh[88] has recently found that in every case in the Mayo Clinic series in which generalized osteitis fibrosa was evident roentgenographically, the alkaline phosphatase was elevated. Conversely, the values were normal in every case in which the diagnosis could not be made roentgenographically. He points out that there is no need to survey the skeleton in any case of hyperparathyroidism in which the alkaline phosphatase values are normal and that the laboratory test is far less costly than the roentgenographic survey.

MINIMAL DIAGNOSTIC CRITERIA

It is not possible to set an arbitrary value for the level of calcium in the serum below which hyperparathyroidism cannot exist. In the Mayo Clinic series, the diagnosis has yet to be made in any case in which the average of several determinations was less than 10.6 mg. per 100 cc. There is no reason to suppose, however, that this value is actually the lower limit of the hypercalcemia of hyperparathyroidism. Average calcium values less than 11 mg. per 100 cc. have been observed in approximately 7 per cent of the cases in the clinic series. Values for serum calcium below

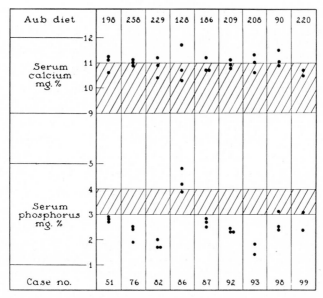

Fig. 16. The values for calcium and phosphorus in serum and the average daily excretion of calcium in the urine on the Aub diet (numbers at top of figure) in nine selected cases of mild hyperparathyroidism.

11 mg. per 100 cc., consequently, cannot be taken as evidence against hyperparathyroidism. The actual values will depend somewhat on the individual laboratory. As previously mentioned, the upper limit of the normal range at the Mayo Clinic is now usually considered to be 10.5 mg. per 100 cc. rather than 11.

In cases in which the hypercalcemia is minimal, the diagnosis usually depends on the values for phosphorus and on excretion studies.[12] The laboratory findings in nine such cases are summarized in Figure 16. In seven of the nine cases the hypercalcemia was associated with definite hypophosphatemia and hypercalciuria. The diagnosis in each of the seven cases seemed established with considerable certainty. In one case (Case 86), the phosphorus values were definitely elevated and the excretion of calcium in the urine was practically normal. Such findings were thought compatible with hyperparathyroidism, since the patient's renal function was moderately impaired. However, the only laboratory evidence for hyperparathyroidism in this case was the hypercalcemia, and the diagnosis consequently was considered somewhat uncertain. In one other case (Case 98) the calcium in the serum was elevated and the phosphorus was depressed, but the urinary excretion was normal. The explanation for this is not clear. Renal function was not greatly impaired as judged by the low values for phosphorus and a value for urea of 34 mg. per 100 cc. of blood. One kidney was functionless, however, and the other was the seat of an infected hydronephrosis, which presumably interfered seriously with the amount of calcium which could be excreted under conditions of the test. The case illustrates the point that hyperparathyroidism may exist without hypercalciuria under the conditions of the Aub diet.

EXCLUSION OF HYPERPARATHYROIDISM

The question of hyperparathyroidism should be raised routinely in all cases of urinary lithiasis. If accurate determinations are available, hyperparathyroidism can be excluded with complete certainty by perhaps two determinations of the calcium and phosphorus in the serum. If the calcium values are 10 mg. per 100 cc. of serum or less and the phosphorus values 3.5 mg. per 100 cc. of serum or more, the urinary stones are not on the basis of hyperparathyroidism and further tests for hyperparathyroidism are not necessary. When consistent values for calcium higher than 10 mg. per 100 cc. are found, further tests, as previously discussed, become necessary. Hypophosphatemia would similarly be an indication for more extended study. Screening tests based on the concentration of calcium in the urine are far less certain than studies of the serum calcium, and should not be relied on either to exclude hyperparathyroidism or to reveal cases in which further studies should be carried out.

While failure to determine the level of calcium in the serum in cases of renal lithiasis is usually responsible for the missed diagnosis, faulty determinations are almost invariably the cause of erroneous diagnosis. The error is made both ways; the incorrect diagnosis is made from erroneously high values, and the correct diagnosis is not established because of erroneously low values. The clinician has some clue to the possibility of faulty determinations if repeated determinations are not reasonably constant.

Chapter VII

DIFFERENTIAL DIAGNOSIS

I F THE differential diagnosis of hyperparathyroidism is approached from the standpoint of the hypercalcemia, which is the one constant laboratory finding in hyperparathyroidism, it immediately becomes much simplified. All types of skeletal disease not characterized by hypercalcemia may be immediately differentiated from the osseous changes of hyperparathyroidism by this one test. Among these may be included osteoporosis, osteomalacia, most cases of Paget's disease, benign giant-cell tumors, multiple solitary cysts of bone, osteogenesis imperfecta, polyostotic fibrous dysplasia, Gaucher's disease, lymphoma, and many others. One variety of osteoporosis, that which follows extensive immobilization of the skeleton or extensive paralysis, particularly in children, may be associated with hypercalcemia, hypercalciuria and even with formation of stones. This type of osteoporosis, in keeping with other types, should present little difficulty in its differentiation from hyperparathyroidism. The cause of the disuse atrophy is evident, the serum phosphorus is not reduced and, most important, the value for alkaline phosphatase is normal and not increased, as it would be if the osseous changes were due to hyperparathyroidism.

Under certain circumstances, Paget's disease may simulate generalized osteitis fibrosa. In the usual case, Paget's disease does not involve all of the skeleton, the serum calcium is normal, as is the serum phosphorus, and the serum phosphatase is higher in proportion to the extent of the osseous disease than in any other condition. If the skeleton involved by Paget's disease is immobilized, bone formation is decreased by the removal of the stresses and strains. The same changes are then found as occur after immobilization of the growing skeleton of childhood. The excretion of calcium and phosphorus in the urine increases. Hypercalcemia develops if the amount of calcium to be excreted exceeds the capacity of the kidneys to dispose of it. Unlike the atrophy of disuse, the alkaline phosphatase is elevated.

In addition to hyperparathyroidism and to cases in which rapid demineralization of the skeleton is occurring just discussed, hypercalcemia occurs in hypervitaminosis D, multiple myeloma, sarcoidosis, osteolytic carcinomatosis, and in the syndrome recently described by Burnett, Commons, Albright and Howard (1949) under the title "Hypercalcemia Without Hypercalcuria or Hypophosphatemia, Calcinosis and Renal Insufficiency; a Syndrome Following Prolonged Intake of Milk and Alkali."

HYPERVITAMINOSIS D

The prolonged administration of massive doses of vitamin D (50,000 units or more per day) may produce changes in the values for calcium and phosphorus in blood and urine which are indistinguishable from those of hyperparathyroidism. Furthermore, the hypercalcemia, hypophosphatemia and hypercalciuria may persist for months after administration of the vitamin has been discontinued. Hyperparathyroidism cannot be excluded with certainty in such cases until possibly six to 12 months after the treatment has been discontinued. Hypervitaminosis D can be excluded only by careful questioning of the patient, and, in some cases, of his medical attendant. There are certain roentgenologic findings, however, which may suggest the correct diagnosis. Prolonged intake of excessive doses of vitamin D may cause metastatic calcification of the soft tissues. The deposits tend to develop in the kidneys, the inner layer of the media or arteries, and particularly in de-vitalized tissues, such as the periarticular soft tissues of patients with rheumatoid arthritis. The deposits have an unusual putty-like appearance. The arterial calcifications appear the same as those of age; in younger persons extensive arterial calcification should suggest the possibility of hypervitaminosis D.

MULTIPLE MYELOMA

While the roentgenographic appearance of the bones in multiple myeloma is usually quite different from that of the skeleton in generalized osteitis fibrosa, the appearance of the bones may be similar. Osseous changes may be absent or may manifest themselves as a solitary tumor or a few punched-out areas. In addition, the serum calcium may be high and there may be hypercalciuria and urinary stones. The serum phosphorus is usually normal but may be reduced. The other clinical features of multiple myeloma are usually sufficient to enable one to establish the correct diagnosis. Bence Jones proteinuria, if present, is strong evidence in favor of myeloma, and examination of the cells secured by sternal puncture is pathognomonic. Furthermore, the value for alkaline phosphatase is normal in myeloma, a point of importance in distinguishing the osseous changes of myeloma from those of generalized osteitis fibrosa.[60]

SARCOIDOSIS

Boeck's sarcoid may rarely be confused with hyperparathyroidism because of osseous changes, high alkaline phosphatase values, hypercalcemia, hypercalciuria and even urinary calculi. The hypercalcemia is often out of proportion to the hyperproteinemia. The increased excretion of calcium in the urine is further evidence that the hypercalcemia is due, in part, to an increase in ionic calcium. The osseous changes are not generalized, however, but limited usually to the hands and feet. The serum phosphatase levels cannot be correlated with the extent of the osseous lesions. The hypercalcemia is not associated with hypophosphatemia. The hyperproteinemia is, in itself, a differential point of some significance. Hyperproteinemia is observed so rarely in hyperparathyroidism that its presence is strong presumptive evidence that some other condition, and not hyperparathyroidism, accounts for the hypercalcemia.

SYNDROME RESULTING FROM PROLONGED AND EXCESSIVE INTAKE OF MILK AND ALKALI

Burnett, Commons, Albright and Howard (1949) reported six cases of a condition resembling hyperparathyroidism with secondary renal damage. The following clinical features were listed: (1) history of prolonged and excessive intake of milk and absorbable alkali; (2) hypercalcemia without hypercalciuria or hypophosphatemia; (3) normal alkaline phosphatase; (4) marked renal insufficiency with azotemia; (5) mild alkalosis; and (6) calcinosis, especially an ocular lesion resembling band keratitis. At least three cases of the same condition have been observed at the Mayo Clinic, in two of which exploration of the parathyroids was carried out. In one case moderate secondary hyperplasia of the parathyroids was found; in the other, the parathyroid glands were considered essentially normal grossly and microscopically. The group at the Mayo Clinic are of the opinion, at the present time, that the syndrome cannot be differentiated with complete certainty from hyperparathyroidism with secondary renal insufficiency in which, usually because of complicating peptic ulcer, the patient has taken large amounts of milk and absorbable alkali. It is admitted that a patient having the syndrome most probably does not have hyperparathyroidism and that the treatment should be a regimen low in calcium and milk with the addition of aluminum gels to decrease absorption of phosphorus. The problem is somewhat academic because of the severe renal damage, which cannot be rectified by any known therapy.

METASTATIC OSTEOLYTIC MALIGNANT GROWTHS

Widespread osteolytic metastatic growths may be associated with hypercalcemia, hypercalciuria and formation of stones. The phosphorus is usually normal but may be elevated or rarely depressed. The phosphatase concentration may be increased. Such changes may occur in the absence of roentgenologic evidence of metastatic growths. The primary carcinoma and other symptoms associated with the malignant lesion or metastatic growths should provide the necessary evidence for the correct diagnosis. Carcinomas of the breast, prostate, kidneys, thyroid and bronchi are most likely to develop widespread osseous metastatic growths.

There is one other diagnostic procedure which may be of value in distinguishing the hypercalcemia of hyperparathyroidism from that due to other causes. Howard and his collaborators (1949) have recently called attention to the fact that neither the low calcium of hypoparathyroidism nor the high calcium of hyperparathyroidism in the serum are reflected by corresponding changes in the level of calcium in the cerebrospinal fluid. Conversely, an increase in the level of diffusible calcium in the serum from other causes is associated with an increase in the calcium of the cerebrospinal fluid. They report that in two cases in which hypercalcemia was due to hyperparathyroidism, the level of calcium in the cerebrospinal fluid was less than the calculated value for the diffusible calcium in serum. In five of six other cases in which the hypercalcemia was on the basis of sarcoid or metastatic malignant lesions, the calcium in the cerebrospinal fluid was elevated and approximately equal to the calculated value for diffusible calcium in the serum. Too few cases have yet been reported to enable one to judge whether the correlation of the level of the calcium in serum with that of the cerebrospinal fluid will prove of practical diagnostic importance.

Chapter VIII

TREATMENT

T HE ONLY known treatment of hyperparathyroidism is surgical removal of the hyperfunctioning tissue. One, more than one, or all of the parathyroid glands may be involved, and an involved gland may be widely aberrant. The lesions may vary greatly in size, a material proportion being so small that their location and recognition are difficult. The immediate aim at operation is the finding of four parathyroid glands. This is far more certain and probably easier than attempting a complete dissection of the widespread region in the neck and upper part of the chest in which parathyroids may be situated. An experienced pathologist, equipped to prepare and diagnose fresh frozen sections, must be available throughout the operation. The question of biopsy will be discussed subsequently, but the pathologist's experience in the field of parathyroid pathology should be such that he can recognize with certainty a parathyroid adenoma, secondary hyperplasia, or primary (wasserhelle) hyperplasia and have a reasonably mature opinion as to atrophy of parathyroid tissue.

The surgeon should be convinced before operation that the patient has hyperparathyroidism and that he must find and remove the offending tissue. He must have the patience and time to carry out a meticulous and often prolonged dissection. He must be sufficiently responsible to appreciate that if a small tumor is missed at the first operation, it will probably never be found, leaving the patient with a potentially fatal but originally curable disease. All secondary operations for hyperparathyroidism are essentially unsatisfactory because of the scarring after the first operation. The practice of carrying out a cursory cervical exploration and of then referring the patient to a surgeon more skilled in the surgery of hyperparathyroidism cannot be too strongly condemned.

The question of removing normal or atrophied glands with the idea of influencing the hyperparathyroidism has long been settled. Such needless sacrifice of parathyroid tissue does not permanently influence hyperparathyroidism and only predisposes the patient to chronic tetany, if and when the tumor is found and removed.

The cervical dissection should be done first, and the mediastinal exploration should be undertaken at a later time. If both mediastinal and cervical explorations are to be carried out at the same sitting, the surgeon, consciously or unconsciously, is likely to be less thorough than if the operative procedure were limited to the cervical region. He is less likely to spend the time and effort necessary to identify each parathyroid gland if he becomes convinced, usually on inadequate grounds, that the tumor is within the mediastinum.

As a final point the question of cure after an apparently fruitless cervical exploration might be mentioned. In one case in the clinic series a cervical dissection was completed without the discovery of any abnormal parathyroid tissue. In addition to hyperparathyroidism, the patient had a nodular goiter which was resected. Subsequent chemical studies demonstrated that the hyperparathyroidism had been cured. It is evident that the postoperative evaluation saved the patient a needless major operation. In some cases, for reasons that are not entirely clear, the calcium level in the blood falls over a period of weeks rather than within a few days after the removal of the hyperfunctioning tissue. In view of this, we now advise that at least three months be allowed to elapse between the cervical and mediastinal explorations. The diagnostic procedures should be again carried out before the final decision to proceed with mediastinal exploration is made.

Before the actual operative procedures are discussed, certain aspects of the surgical anatomy and surgical pathology will be reviewed. Before attempting to treat hyperparathyroidism, the surgeon should have developed the ability to recognize parathyroid glands, and should be thoroughly cognizant with the variations in lesions causing hyperparathyroidism and with the varied locations of the parathyroid glands.

NORMAL PARATHYROID GLANDS

Many opinions to the contrary, a normal parathyroid gland is rather easily recognizable grossly. Unless situated in loose areolar tissue, when it is globular, the gland is flattened or stretched and appears as an ovoid plate or disk. It may be piriform or leaflike and often contains small cysts.[27] It is softer than a lymph node and much softer than thyroid tissue. The usual dimensions are approximately 6 by 4 by 1.5 mm., and the average weight is 30 to 40 mg.[53] The most characteristic feature of a parathyroid gland of an adult is the yellow-brown color. Thyroid tissue is far redder, lymph nodes are much lighter and pinker, and thymic tissue is a much paler yellow color. In the newborn the glands are gray and semitransparent; the yellowish cast appears first at from six to 10 years of age; the adult appearance is achieved at from 11 to 20 years of age.[31] There is a definite though delicate capsule, through which a network of subcapsular vessels may be seen. The gland is more or less enclosed in a small pad of fat, which, however, does not obscure the characteristic color. The fatty pad is often thickened at one or both poles, giving the appearance of a fatty halo. The color, the smooth surface, the reticulum of vessels beneath the capsule and the fatty pad all help in identification.

Each parathyroid gland is supplied by a single small artery which enters at a definite hilus.[61] If the gland is situated in the capsule of the thyroid the vascular pedicle is not striking. In those cases in which the gland is situated at a distance from the thyroid, the pedicle is more definite. The arterial supply of the superior pair of glands in all cases comes from the inferior thyroid artery or from the anastomotic channel between the inferior and superior thyroid arteries. This is also true in the great majority of inferior glands. Widely aberrant inferior glands may derive their blood supply indifferently from the nearest arterial source.[109]

ATROPHIC PARATHYROID GLANDS

With hyperparathyroidism, atrophy of the uninvolved glands is to be expected, and the finding of an atrophic gland is further evidence that the diagnosis of hyperparathyroidism is correct. In some cases, on the other hand, uninvolved glands may appear normal, so that the finding of an apparently normal gland should not be taken as evidence against the diagnosis. An atrophic gland is far more difficult to recognize than a normal gland, chiefly because of the progressive loss of the characteristic brownish color as the gland becomes atrophic. There is less change in the size of the gland than would be anticipated. About half of the bulk of a normal gland is parenchyma, and about half is fat-containing stroma. With the development of atrophy the fatty stroma increases at the expense of the parenchyma so that there may be little over-all change in size. The characteristic color, on the other hand, becomes progressively less distinctive as the yellow color of the fatty stroma dilutes the darker brown of the parenchyma. With experience, it is still usually possible to identify the atrophic gland grossly with some certainty because of the persistence of some of the brownish color and through the unchanged general architecture of fatty pad, capsule, subcapsular vessels and vascular pedicle.

NUMBER OF GLANDS

The careful dissections of Gilmour (1938) have largely solved the problem of the number of the parathyroid glands. Both Sandstrom (1880) and Welsh (1898) were able to find four glands in the great majority of their dissections, but their findings were obscured by the supposed finding of as many as from six to 12 glands by others. Gilmour found a total of 1,713 glands in 428 necropsy cases, or an average of four glands per case. Two glands only were found in one case and three glands in 26 cases, or 6.1 per cent. When fewer than four glands were found, the total weight suggested that in most cases a gland had been missed in the dissection. Rarely the two glands on one side were fused, a condition described first by Welsh (1898). It was concluded that cases in which there were fewer than four glands must be accepted, but that such cases were decidedly unusual. Five glands were found in 25 cases (6 per cent) and six glands in two cases. As a rule when more than four glands were found, the supernumerary glands were small, and usually lay close to a gland of normal size. These findings support the conception that, for practical purposes, the possibility of more than four glands in aberrant locations need not greatly disturb the surgeon operating for hyperparathyroidism.

LOCATION OF PARATHYROID GLANDS

The varied locations of parathyroid glands are due principally to their embryonic development.[28] The superior pair of glands (parathyroid IV, true parathyroids) develop in close association with the lateral anlagen of the thyroid from the fourth pharyngeal pouch. They early assume a position on the dorsal and medial surface of the corresponding developing thyroid lobe, and usually are found, in the adult, at about the junction of the middle and upper thirds of the lobe (Fig. 1). Their medial position was early stressed by Welsh (1898), who described them as lying on the hypopharynx or esophagus rather than on the thyroid. The region in which a superior gland may be found is more limited than that of an inferior gland. It is bounded above by the upper border of the larynx, or well above the superior pole of the thyroid, inferiorly by the lower pole of the thyroid, anteriorly by the middle layer of the deep cervical fascia and posteriorly by the prevertebral fascia. The medial and lateral boundaries are the hypopharynx or esophagus and the carotid sheath respectively. Glands may be situated behind the esophagus or within the carotid sheath. Gilmour (1938) found more than 90 per cent of superior glands on the posterior or medial surface of the thyroid, above the lower third.

The inferior pair of glands (parathyroid III, parathymus) develop rostrad to the superior glands from the third pharyngeal pouch, in close association with the anlagen of the thymus. The developing gland "descends" with the thymus along a course anterior and lateral to that of the ipsilateral superior gland and usually comes to lie near the inferior pole of the thyroid gland anterolaterally as well as caudally to the superior gland. The adult gland is usually in one of three positions in relation to the inferior pole of the thyroid: (1) closely associated with the capsule of the thyroid just anterior to the terminal branches of the inferior thyroid artery; (2) in about the same plane but caudal to the inferior pole; and (3) caudal to the inferior pole but nearer the trachea, closely associated with the inferior thyroid veins. The inferior gland may be found, however, in the visceral compartment of the cervical fascia at any level from above the superior pole of the thyroid rostrally to beneath the arch of the aorta caudally. The gland is often intimately associated with a small mass of thymic tissue and, in the mediastinum, may be within the thymus. In Gilmour's series, approximately 95 per cent of the inferior glands were in the immediate vicinity of the lower poles of the thyroid. In another 3 per cent of cases the glands were between 3 to 6 cm. distal to the inferior pole, but in one case, not included in the series, one inferior gland was 9 cm. and the other 11 cm. below the poles of the thyroid. One inferior gland only in the series was above the superior pole.

In addition to the embryologic displacement described previously, an adult gland, particularly when enlarged, may be displaced caudally by the same forces which cause thyroid adenomas to sink into the thorax. A superior gland, because of its dorsal position, tends to descend into the posterior superior mediastinum. An inferior gland, depending on its original position, may descend into either the anterior or the posterior superior mediastinum. A cervical gland displaced into the mediastinum carried its blood supply with it and consequently has a pedicle which connects the gland with the vascular supply of the thyroid, usually the inferior thyroid artery. A gland which develops in the mediastinum may receive its blood supply from any neighboring vessel and may not have a pedicle leading into the cervical region. On this basis, all parathyroid glands in the posterior superior mediastinum have vascular pedicles extending into the cervical region. Those in the anterior superior mediastinum may or may not have pedicles.

Any of the parathyroid glands may be incorporated within the corresponding lobe of the thyroid gland. The earlier skepticism concerning intrathyroidal parathyroid tissue was based, principally, on failure to find parathyroid glands within the thyroid by gross dissection. In addition, none of the adenomas in the Mayo Clinic series nor in the Massachusetts General Hospital series through 1947 had been found within the thyroid.[23] Norris (1947) however, reported that approximately 3 per cent of the adenomas reported in the literature had been situated within the thyroid. Since 1947, two intrathyroidal adenomas have been found at the Mayo Clinic, so that approximately 2 per cent of parathyroid adenomas in the series have been intrathyroidal.[24] In each case the possibility that the adenoma was merely situated deeply in a sulcus of the thyroid seemed to be excluded with reasonable certainty.

LOCATION OF PARATHYROID ADENOMAS

An adenoma obviously may develop in parathyroid tissue wherever situated. In the great majority of cases the adenomas are situated in the immediate vicinity of the thyroid gland. In the 281 cases collected from the literature by Norris (1947), only 30 adenomas were aberrant—that is, were not closely associated with the thyroid gland—and 19 only were within the mediastinum. Of 58 adenomas in Cope's[38] series 11 were within the anterior mediastinum and five were in the posterior mediastinum. The cervical region had been explored previously in nine cases. Of the nine, the adenoma was found in the anterior mediastinum in six cases and in the posterior mediastinum in one case. In the 49 cases in which operation had not been performed previously, five adenomas were found in the anterior mediastinum and four in the posterior mediastinum. Considering Norris' and Cope's series together it would appear that in only about 10 per cent of cases were the adenomas within the mediastinum.

This does not imply that exploration of the anterior superior mediastinum will be necessary in 10 per cent of cases of hyperparathyroidism due to adenomas. All adenomas in the posterior superior mediastinum should be accessible through the cervical incision since they are never deeply placed within the chest. They are virtually never large enough to be forced further into the chest by their own growth, and there is no large cervical goiter to force them downward as is the case with certain intrathoracic goiters. Similarly, many adenomas in the anterior superior mediastinum are just within the chest and may be safely removed under direct vision from the cervical approach. In the remaining cases in which the adenoma is in the anterior superior or anterior mediastinum, the adenoma develops in mediastinal parathyroid glands and may be situated some distance below the superior strait of the chest. Anterior mediastinotomy is necessary to expose such deeply placed adenomas.

In the Mayo Clinic series of 102 cases of single or multiple adenomas there was a total of 106 adenomas. Four adenomas were well within the anterior superior mediastinum and not immediately apparent on cervical dissection. In two of the four cases the adenoma was found and removed under direct vision through the cervical incision. In both cases the adenomas were found because of a well-defined vascular pedicle leading into the mediastinum from the cervical region (Fig. 17). In the remaining two cases, formal exploration of the anterior superior mediastinum through a sternotomy incision was necessary to expose the adenoma. If the series is representative, exploration of the anterior superior mediastinum should rarely

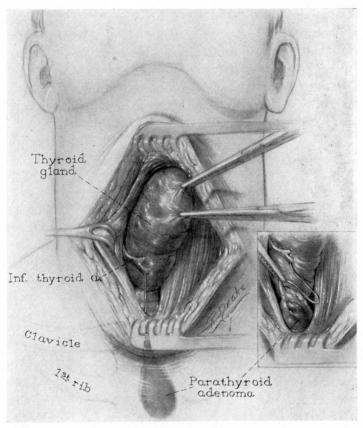

Fig. 17. Intrathoracic adenoma found and removed through a cervical incision. The vascular pedicle extending into the chest from the inferior thyroid artery is well shown.

be necessary (less than 2 per cent of cases). Before terminating a fruitless cervical dissection, the surgeon should appreciate, to quote the extremes reported in the literature, that there is only from one chance in 10 to one chance in 50 that mediastinal exploration is actually necessary to reveal the adenoma.

SIZE OF PARATHYROID ADENOMAS

Because of the frequent distortion of adenomas, size will be discussed in terms of weight rather than dimension. In the Mayo Clinic series, the adenomas weighed less than 100 mg. in 3 per cent of cases, less than 500 mg. in 22 per cent of cases, and less than 1 gm. in 34 per cent of cases. The tumors weighed between 1 and 5 gm. in 30 per cent of cases and more than 10 gm. in less than 10 per cent of cases. The preponderance of small tumors in the Mayo Clinic series is at sharp variance with the size of tumors in the series of cases collected from the literature by Norris (1947). Considering only those in which weight had been reported, there were none in the collected series which weighed less than 200 mg., and 5 per cent only weighed less than 1 gm. Slightly more than 35 per cent weighed between 1 and 5 gm., 20 per cent between 5 and 10 gm. and almost 40 per cent more than 10 gm.

The apparent difference between the two series can be easily resolved. In practically all cases in the collected series, skeletal disease was present. Demineralization of bones is far more likely to occur in the presence of severe hypercalcemia and hypercalciuria than in cases with a less marked negative calcium balance. Consequently, the collected series could be described more accurately as cases of generalized osteitis fibrosa than as cases of hyperparathyroidism in general. In the cases of hyperparathyroidism complicated by osteitis fibrosa in the Mayo Clinic series, the mean size of the adenoma was 5.6 gm., even excluding the one case in which the tumor weighed 101 gm. This mean weight is in close agreement with the mean weight of 7 gm. in the collected series. The mean level of calcium in the serum in cases of osteitis fibrosa at the clinic was 14.6 mg. per 100 cc. while the corresponding value in cases without osseous disease was 12 mg. The tumors in the group without evidence of osseous disease had a mean weight of 1.6 gm. There are, unfortunately, many exceptions to the generalization that large adenomas are to be expected in cases of generalized osteitis fibrosa and small tumors in cases of hyperparathyroidism without bone disease. The second smallest tumor in the Mayo Clinic series, which weighed, along with some surrounding fat, 54 mg., had caused classic generalized osteitis fibrosa.

Some knowledge of the expected size of the adenoma would obviously be of great help to the surgeon. As previously intimated when the size of the adenoma, the level of serum calcium and the presence of skeletal disease were mentioned, there is a crude correlation between the size of the adenoma and the value for calcium in the serum. Larger adenomas may be expected in cases in which the level of calcium is high, and small adenomas when the hypercalcemia is minimal. The problem of size was less important during the years when only patients who had generalized osteitis fibrosa were treated surgically. It has become increasingly important since the diagnosis has become possible in cases with minimal hypercalcemia. Adenomas larger than 1 gm. are usually easily found; those which weigh less than 1 gm. are not only less evident but are likely to be caught in sulci of the thyroid or, more usually, in tissue spaces between contiguous structures and so concealed. The small size of many adenomas causes as much difficulty surgically as aberrant location.

The relationship between the weight of the adenoma and the level of calcium in the serum in those cases in the Mayo Clinic series in which the weight is known is shown in Figure 18. Tumors which weighed less than 2 gm. were compared to those which weighed 2 gm. or more. With this division there were approximately an equal number of cases in the two groups. In the case of the smaller tu-

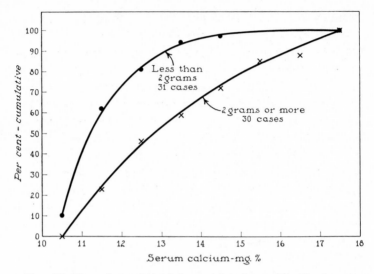

Fig. 18. The relationship of the weight of parathyroid adenomas to the level of serum calcium. Adenomas which weighed less than 2 gm. were compared with those which weighed 2 gm. or more. In 60 per cent of the smaller tumors, the calcium values were less than 12 mg. per 100 cc. of serum whereas in fewer than 25 per cent of the larger tumors were calcium values so low.

mors (less than 2 gm.), the serum calcium was between 10 and 11 mg. per 100 cc. in 10 per cent of cases, and in 60 per cent of the cases the calcium value was less than 12 mg. In the case of the larger adenomas (2 gm. or more in weight) there were none with calcium values less than 11 mg., and fewer than 25 per cent with values less than 12. The following approximations were also possible from the study of the group. In those cases in which the value for calcium was less than 12 mg. per 100 cc. of serum, one third of the adenomas weighed less than 0.5 gm., one third between 0.5 and 1 gm. and one third more than 1 gm. In cases in which the calcium values were between 12 and 14 mg. per 100 cc. of serum, one third of the adenomas weighed less than 1 gm. and two thirds more than 1 gm. In cases in which the value for calcium was 14 mg. or more per 100 cc. of serum, the adenoma weighed less than 1 gm. in fewer than 10 per cent of cases.

The range of the weights of adenomas for all values of calcium greater than 11 mg. per 100 cc. of serum, however, was so great that, apart from the general trend, little concerning the size of the tumor could be predicted from the value for serum calcium. Thus, with calcium values between 11 and 12 mg. per 100 cc. of serum, the adenomas varied in weight from less than 100 mg. to more than 10 gm., and even with values as high as 17 to 18 mg. per 100 cc. of serum, the size of the tumor varied from 1 gm. to more than 10 gm.

Chapter IX

SURGICAL PROCEDURES

CERVICAL DISSECTION

S INCE the dissection is to be carried out in the immediate vicinity of the recurrent laryngeal nerves, local anesthesia using 0.5 per cent solution of procaine as a field
block, augmented by nitrous oxide and oxygen, is em-
ployed. If there is justification for such anesthesia in thyroid surgery, it is doubly justified in parathyroid surgery
because of the much greater risk of nerve injuries. It must
be admitted that a prolonged dissection under local and
light general anesthesia is far more trying to both the patient and the surgeon than is general anesthesia using an
intratracheal tube. The choice of anesthesia, like most of
the details of the surgical treatment of hyperparathyroidism, has not become standardized. General anesthesia is
preferred by some.

The incision, the elevation of skin flaps and the division
in the midline of the fused superficial and middle layer of
the deep cervical fascia are carried out as in performing a
thyroidectomy. Beneath the plane of the cervical fascia the
staining of tissues with blood is avoided at all cost.

Since the operation is to be bilateral and since there is
as much chance of pathologic tissue on one side as on the
other, it makes little difference which lobe of the thyroid
is first elevated. The chosen lobe is elevated and rotated
extensively. The areolar tissue is carefully cleared from
around the lobe, the superior and inferior thyroid arteries
and the inferior thyroid veins. The inferior thyroid artery
is found and is usually ligated. The recurrent laryngeal
nerve is exposed from its entrance into the operative field

to the adherent zone of the thyroid. After these preliminary steps a careful search is instituted for first the superior and then the inferior parathyroid gland. Gross identification of the atrophic glands is adequate at this stage of the procedure. If the uninvolved glands are atrophic, which is to be expected, gross identification will be uncertain. The dangers of destroying the atrophied gland or its blood supply by removing tissue for biopsy is so great that all biopsies should be avoided until they become mandatory at a later stage of a fruitless exploration.

As the final step of this phase of the procedure the areolar tissue is cleaned widely from the carotid arteries and jugular veins, and the dissection is carried distally under direct vision into the posterior superior mediastinum. The patient is awakened in order to determine the integrity of the recurrent laryngeal nerve. The same procedure is then carried out on the opposite side of the neck.

The procedure from this stage on depends on the findings, or lack of findings. In the usual case an adenoma will have been encountered and the dissection will have been sufficiently extended to exclude with reasonable certainty a second adenoma. The complete removal of the adenoma would then finish the operation. Tetany was so feared formerly, particularly in cases with extensive osseous disease and high alkaline phosphatase values, after complete removal of an adenoma, that subtotal resection was often carried out. The practice has been abandoned, since tetany can now be treated successfully. As discussed previously, the cytologic character of many adenomas may be so similar to that of adenocarcinomas that the exact pathologic classification is often doubtful. This being so, total removal of all parathyroid tumors in all cases is necessary to avoid partial removal of a carcinoma.

In cases in which the preliminary bilateral dissection has

failed to reveal an adenoma, biopsies become necessary in order to identify with certainty each of the parathyroid glands provisionally identified grossly. The biopsies must be made with extreme caution to avoid complete destruction of the gland. The finding of fat only in the specimen does not imply that the nodule under suspicion is not a parathyroid gland, since only a portion of the fatty capsule may have been removed. In this case another minute bit of tissue should be removed. This method of removing multiple tiny specimens for biopsy is most time-consuming, but it is quite necessary if the gland is to be identified with certainty without destroying it in the process of securing tissue for biopsy. As soon as a positive biopsy has been secured the same process is repeated on the next gland. If a gland cannot be found, the dissection is extended to include the entire region in the neck in which the gland may theoretically be situated.

At the conclusion of the complete cervical dissection, in those cases in which the adenoma is actually within the anterior superior mediastinum, three of the four parathyroids should have been identified. While this ideal may be impossible to achieve, it is nevertheless a measure of the completeness of the cervical dissection. In no other way can the surgeon be certain that an adenoma in the cervical region has not been missed.

Vascular pedicles leading into the mediastinum from the vascular system of the thyroid should be carefully sought (Fig. 17). The arterial twig may be surprisingly large. It usually leaves the inferior thyroid artery or the anastomotic channel between superior and inferior thyroid arteries very close to the thyroid. In a careful dissection the pedicle should have become apparent, if present, at some time during the earlier stages of the dissection. The pedicle should be traced into the mediastinum under direct vision before one resorts to biopsies and possible destruc-

tion of uninvolved glands. As previously discussed, all
adenomas within the posterior superior mediastinum theoretically should have pedicles from the cervical region.
Adenomas within the anterior superior mediastinum may
or may not have such pedicles.

As a final step in a cervical dissection which has been
fruitless up to this point each lobe of the thyroid gland
should be carefully examined and occasionally even in-
cised to exclude intrathyroidal parathyroid adenomas. Possibly 2 to 3 per cent of parathyroid adenomas develop
within the thyroid gland. In both cases in the Mayo Clinic
series, the intrathyroidal adenomas were situated within
the lower pole of the thyroid, which was somewhat larger,
and in retrospect, had a slight brownish cast compared
to other parts of the thyroid. It is not unusual to carry
out a subtotal thyroidectomy as the concluding step in
the dissection if a goiter is present.

In the usual case of primary parathyroid hyperplasia
relatively large masses of coffee-brown tissue are encountered on either side, lateral to and behind the thyroid.
Unless the hyperplastic tissue is so extensive that it interferes with the dissection, no tissue should be resected
until the full extent of the hyperplastic tissue has been
determined. After the masses have been freed from surrounding tissues one can be more certain of preserving
vascularized tissue than if the hyperplastic tissue is removed as it is encountered. Sprague and I recently reviewed all previously reported cases with reference to the
amount of hyperplastic tissue which had been preserved.
Tetany had not resulted when as little as 30 mg. (estimated
weight) had been saved, and hyperparathyroidism had
not persisted when as much as 200 mg. had been left behind. It would thus seem that from 30 to 200 mg. of viable
tissue should be preserved in such cases.

Primary hyperplasia, in rare cases, may not be apparent as such grossly. In such cases one gland may be greatly enlarged while the others show little, if any, gross hypertrophy. Since adenomas may be composed almost exclusively of wasserhelle cells, a biopsy from the enlarged gland may be incorrectly interpreted as a wasserhelle-cell adenoma. The correct pathologic interpretation is greatly facilitated by a biopsy from one of the apparently uninvolved glands. The practice, in fact, of removing a specimen for biopsy from one gland in addition to removing the tumor is advisable in most cases of hyperparathyroidism.

If an infiltrating carcinoma is found, the tumor theoretically should be removed as radically as possible. The contiguous thyroid tissue, or even the entire lobe, possibly the recurrent laryngeal nerve and all accessible regional lymph nodes, should be sacrificed. It must be admitted that surgical efforts to cure infiltrating carcinoma of parathyroid origin have met with little or no success. However, in practically all cases so far reported, the first resection was limited and not a radical procedure. In cases in which the tumor is still confined to the capsule, local complete removal is still generally practiced, apparently successfully, regardless of the immediate pathologic interpretation.

MEDIASTINAL DISSECTION

As discussed previously, surgical exploration of the anterior superior mediastinum is necessary in probably less than 5 per cent of cases. We agree with Cope[38] (1941) that the dissection of the mediastinum should be done as a separate procedure and not in conjunction with the cervical dissection, as recently proposed by Rienhoff (1949). We prefer to delay the dissection for three months and to verify the diagnosis by chemical determinations before opening the chest. The adenoma may be just within the mediastinum or it may be as low as the pericardium. It is usually in the same plane as the thymus and may be within the thymus.[1] It may also be in the plane of the great veins.

Positive pressure anesthesia using an intratracheal tube is necessary. The same approach is used as that for thymectomy.[34, 38] The incision in the skin extends from the healed incision of the cervical dissection to the xyphoid. The scarring in the manubrial notch and that behind the upper part of the manubrium resulting from the previous cervical dissection is opened into by blunt and sharp dissection. A finger is then inserted behind the manubrium, separating the soft tissues from the bone. A Lebsche sternal chisel is inserted, and the manubrium and sternum are split in the midline from the sternal notch to the xyphoid. The manubrium is rather dense and splits with greater difficulty than the body. Some bleeding from the sternal marrow is to be expected. A self-retaining retractor is inserted, and the split sternum is spread to expose the anterior mediastinum.

As in the cervical operation, the dissection must be meticulous and bleeding must be avoided. The fat and areolar tissue of the mediastinum are separated from the thymus and vessels. The blood supply of the thymus is fairly constant and can usually be largely avoided. The arterial supply from the inferior thyroid arteries enters the upward projections of the thymus on either side and that from the internal mammary arteries joins the thymus on either side at about the level of the isthmus joining the two lobes. The venous drainage is by one or two vessels which pass directly backward from the posterior surface of the isthmus to the left innominate vein. The mediastinal pleura, which is most delicate, is pushed carefully aside.

The dissection should be carried proximally into the

region of scarring resulting from the cervical operation. The majority of adenomas will be high in the mediastinum and closely associated with the upward prolongations of the thymus. However, much lower adenomas have been reported. If the dissection of the mediastinum fails to reveal an adenoma, the thymus should be removed. The thymus is friable and should be handled carefully. After the thymus has been removed the pulmonary artery, the arch of the aorta and its branches, the left innominate vein and the pericardium are exposed. Adenomas situated deep to the thymus may not be apparent until the thymus has been removed.

The split sternum is closed by interrupted sutures through the periosteum and fascia on the anterior surface of the bone. The subcutaneous tissues and skin are each closed by a separate row of sutures. If either pleural space has been opened no attempt is made to close the delicate mediastinal pleura. Air is aspirated by means of a catheter while the anesthetist keeps the lung expanded with positive pressure during the closure. No drains are used.

Chapter X

POSTOPERATIVE COURSE AND COMPLICATIONS

WITH the exception of hypophosphatemia, the metabolic changes which characterize hyperparathyroidism revert toward normal rather promptly after removal of the hyperfunctioning tissue. The increased values for serum calcium decline to normal or subnormal levels within 24 to 48 hours (Fig. 19, curve 2), and there is a corresponding decrease in the excretion of calcium in the urine. Keating, Sprague and Power found that phosphorus virtually disappeared from the urine during the first 72 hours after operation and was present thereafter in the urine in decreased amounts. The return of the phosphorus values in the serum to normal may require far more time than that required for the calcium to fall to the normal level. In many cases, phosphorus values remain depressed for weeks or even months after operation.

As previously mentioned, there is definite oliguria during the first 24 hours after operation. The oliguria results from the sudden withdrawal of the excess parathyroid hormone, which has a diuretic effect. The oliguria, theoretically, would favor the deposition of calcium in the tubules or the development of stones. It should be countered by giving 2 or 3 liters of fluids parenterally during the early postoperative period.

Some symptoms of tetany are to be expected postoperatively. In cases in which there is no skeletal disease, the tetany is usually mild and rarely requires treatment. The symptoms are due, in part, to the abrupt decrease in the concentration of ionic calcium in the serum, and, in part,

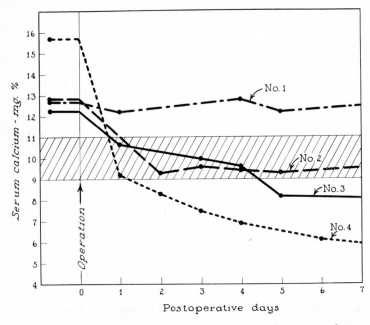

Fɪɢ. 19. Preoperative and postoperative values for serum calcium in 4 cases of hyperparathyroidism. Curve 1: No change in calcium after removal of one adenoma; persisting hyperparathyroidism in case of multiple parathyroid adenomas. Curve 2: Usual change in serum calcium after removal of single adenoma. Cure. Curve 3: Chronic tetany after inadvertent removal or destruction of all parathyroid tissue. Curve 4: Bone-hunger tetany. Severe osseous disease. Alkaline phosphatase 38 Bodansky units. Level of calcium fell to less than 6 mg. per 100 cc. of serum despite all treatment. As skeleton recalcified tetany disappeared.

to the decline of the level of calcium in the serum to the tetanic range. The hypocalcemia results from hypofunction of the atrophic parathyroid glands. It is temporary, usually persisting for a few days only, when the symptoms disappear and the level of calcium tends to rise (Fig. 19, curve 2). Tetany may fail to develop in patients with acidosis due to impaired renal function.

True parathyroprival tetany is unusual, but it does

occur occasionally despite all precautions. There is always some danger of destroying uninvolved parathyroid glands or their blood supply during the necessarily extensive dissections. An atrophic gland is particularly jeopardized by biopsy and consequently biopsies should be avoided whenever possible. Atrophic glands should never be removed, since the procedure does not influence the hyperparathyroidism and only predisposes the patient to tetany when the adenoma is ultimately found and removed. In cases in which all parathyroid tissue has been destroyed, the level of calcium in the serum does not return toward normal as it does in cases in which one or more glands have been saved (Fig. 19, curve 3). The symptoms become progressively worse and treatment becomes mandatory. Treatment should not be delayed until symptoms are extreme. The development of carpopedal spasm or convulsions indicates that treatment is long overdue. Treatment should probably be started in any case in which there is more than a minimal Chvostek sign and numbness or tingling of the hands and feet.

Except as an emergency measure and in cases of bone-hunger tetany, discussed subsequently, there is little place for either intravenously administered calcium or parathyroid extract in the treatment of chronic tetany. However, sterile ampules of calcium chloride (10-20 cc. of 5 per cent solution) or of calcium gluconate (10 cc. of 20 per cent solution) should be instantly available if convulsions are imminent. A single ampule given intravenously usually relieves all symptoms promptly and may be repeated within an hour or so. The effect of parathyroid extract is usually not apparent for several hours but lasts for some 20 hours. The extract is given intramuscularly in doses of from 100 to 500 units. The level of calcium in the serum must be followed closely to avoid overdosage. The effect tends to be lost on repeated dosage. Since better and less expensive methods are available, the extract is little used.

The treatment of choice is calcium given orally combined with dihydrotachysterol (A.T.10; hytakerol®). Calcium lactate or gluconate is prepared by dissolving in boiling water. The usual starting dose is from 32 to 48 gm. per day. This is given in conjunction with dihydrotachysterol, up to 3 cc. per day. As soon as the level of the calcium has been elevated, the amounts of both calcium and dihydrotachysterol are decreased. In the usual case 12 to 16 gm. of calcium lactate and 1 cc. of dihydrotachysterol every other day or every third day will maintain the level of serum calcium within normal limits. The Sulkowitch test may be used to regulate dosage. This is usually not necessary, however, once the maintenance dose has been established. Vitamin D, in doses of from 50,000 to 100,000 units or even more, may be used in place of the dihydrotachysterol.[80] The action of dihydrotachysterol simulates more closely that of parathyroid hormone than does that of vitamin D. However, the effects of vitamin D are more lasting and it is slightly less expensive than dihydrotachysterol.

Another type of tetany, described by Albright as bone-hunger tetany, develops only in those cases with osseous disease and high alkaline phosphatase values. If the alkaline phosphatase level is greater than 20 Bodansky units, severe tetany, requiring far more aggressive treatment than that previously outlined, is to be expected postoperatively (Fig. 19, curve 4). In the past, in cases with extensive osseous disease, subtotal resection of adenomas was often practiced. With greater experience in the management of such conditions, and particularly with the advent of dihydrotachysterol, the practice has been abandoned. The tetany results from the rapid remineralization of the skeleton, which depletes the serum of calcium. To maintain an adequate calcium level in the serum, massive doses of calcium by mouth and even by vein along with large amounts of dihydrotachysterol or of vitamin D are required. Such cases must be managed on an individual basis, and intensive treatment may be required for months before the skeleton has become remineralized.

Except for tetany and oliguria, the postoperative complications do not differ from those after other cervical or anterior mediastinal operations. Paralysis of the vocal cords is perhaps commoner than after thyroidectomy because much of the dissection is carried out in the immediate vicinity of the recurrent laryngeal nerves. The combination of one fixed vocal cord and tetany may be associated with stridor, which can be relieved by the intravenous injection of 10 cc. of 20 per cent solution of calcium gluconate. The stridor may of course recur when the level of calcium in the serum again falls. If the stridor is not relieved immediately, tracheotomy should be considered.

In cases in which there is skeletal disease with severe pain, pathologic fractures should be guarded against, particularly during the first month or so after operation. The skeletal pains tend to disappear long before the skeleton has become recalcified. The lack of pain encourages the patient to move about more freely and exposes him to a greater chance of sustaining a fracture. The danger is further magnified by the fact that unfamiliar crutches or a cane may be used.

The ultimate outcome of treatment depends on the extent of damage to the kidneys. Beyond a certain point, renal impairment is probably progressive, in spite of cure of the hyperparathyroidism, and the patient dies of renal insufficiency or hypertension. Hyperparathyroidism caused by adenomas and wasserhelle hyperplasia does not recur. That caused by infiltrating or metastasized carcinoma almost invariably recurs and ultimately causes death.

REFERENCES

1. ABRAMS, M., RUTENBURG, A. M., LESSES, M. F. and GARGILL, S. L.: Hyperparathyroidism with Nephrolithiasis; Report of a Case with a Parathyroid Tumor Located Within the Thymus. *New England J. Med.*, **241**:401-406 (Sept. 15) 1949.

2. ALBRIGHT, FULLER: Hyperparathyroidism: Its Diagnosis and Exclusion. *New England J. Med.*, **209**:476-480 (Sept. 7) 1933.

3. ALBRIGHT, FULLER: The Parathyroids—Physiology and Therapeutics. *J.A.M.A.*, **117**:527-533 (Aug. 16) 1941.

4. ALBRIGHT, FULLER: Page Out of History of Hyperparathyroidism. *J. Clin. Endocrinol.*, **8**:637-657 (Aug.) 1948.

5. ALBRIGHT, FULLER, AUB, J. C. and BAUER, WALTER: Hyperparathyroidism. A Common and Polymorphic Condition as Illustrated by Seventeen Proved Cases from One Clinic. *J.A.M.A.*, **102**:1276-1287 (Apr. 21) 1934.

6. ALBRIGHT, FULLER, BAIRD, P. C., COPE, OLIVER and BLOOMBERG, ESTHER: Studies on the Physiology of the Parathyroid Glands. IV. Renal Complications of Hyperparathyroidism. *Am. J. M. Sc.*, **187**:49-65 (Jan.) 1934.

7. ALBRIGHT, FULLER, BAUER, WALTER, ROPES, MARION and AUB, J. C.: Studies of Calcium and Phosphorus Metabolism. IV. The Effect of the Parathyroid Hormone. *J. Clin. Investigation,* **7**:139-181 (Apr.) 1929.

8. ALBRIGHT, FULLER, BLOOMBERG, ESTHER, CASTLEMAN, BENJAMIN and CHURCHILL, E. D.: Hyperparathyroidism Due to Diffuse Hyperplasia of all Parathyroid Glands Rather Than Adenoma of One: Clinical Studies on Three Such Cases. *Arch. Int. Med.*, **54**:315-329 (Sept.) 1934.

9. ALBRIGHT, FULLER, BURNETT, C. H., PARSON, WILLIAM, REIFENSTEIN, E. C., JR. and ROOS, ALBERT: Osteomalacia and Late Rickets; the Various Etiologies Met in the United States with Emphasis on That Resulting from a Specific

Form of Renal Acidosis, the Therapeutic Indications for Each Etiological Sub-group, and the Relationship Between Osteomalacia and Milkman's Syndrome. *Medicine*, **25**:399-479 (Dec.) 1946.

10. ALBRIGHT, FULLER and ELLSWORTH, READ: Studies on the Physiology of the Parathyroid Glands. I. Calcium and Phosphorus Studies on a Case of Idiopathic Hypoparathyroidism. *J. Clin. Investigation*, **7**:183-201 (June) 1929.

11. ALBRIGHT, FULLER and REIFENSTEIN, E. C., JR.: *Parathyroid Glands and Metabolic Bone Disease*. Baltimore, Williams & Wilkins Company, 1948, pp. 15, 73.

12. ALBRIGHT, FULLER, SULKOWITCH, H. W. and BLOOMBERG, ESTHER: Further Experience in the Diagnosis of Hyperparathyroidism, Including a Discussion of Cases with a Minimal Degree of Hyperparathyroidism. *Am. J. M. Sc.*, **193**:800-812 (June) 1937.

13. ALBRIGHT, F., SULKOWITCH, H. W. and BLOOMBERG, E.: Hyperparathyroidism Due to Idiopathic Hypertrophy (Hyperplasia?) of Parathyroid Tissue; Follow-up Report of six Cases. *Arch. Int. Med.*, **62**:199-215 (Aug.) 1938.

14. ALEXANDER, H. B., PEMBERTON, J. DEJ., KEPLER, E. J. and BRODERS, A. C.: Functional Parathyroid Tumors and Hyperparathyroidism: Clinical and Pathologic Considerations. *Am. J. Surg.*, n.s. **65**:157-188 (Aug.) 1944.

15. ANSPACH, W. E. and CLIFTON, W. M.: Hyperparathyroidism in Children; Report of Two Cases. *Am. J. Dis. Child.*, **58**:540-557 (Sept.) 1939.

16. ASKANAZY, M.: Ueber Ostitis deformans ohne osteides Gewebe. *Arb. a. d. Geb. d. path. Anat. Inst. zu Tübingen.*, **4**:398-422, 1904.

17. BARNEY, J. D. and SULKOWITCH, H. W.: Progress in the Management of Urinary Calculi. *J. Urol.*, **37**:746-762 (June) 1937.

18. BARR, D. P., BULGER, H. A. and DIXON, H. H.: Hyperparathyroidism. *J.A.M.A.*, **92**:951-952 (Mar. 23) 1929.

19. BAUER, WALTER and AUB, J. C.: Studies of Inorganic Salt

Metabolism. I. The Ward Routine and Methods. *J. Am. Dietet. A.*, **3**:106-115 (Sept.) 1927.

20. BEARD, D. E. and GOODYEAR, W. E.: Hyperparathyroidism and Urolithiasis. *J. Urol.*, **64**:638-642 (Nov.) 1950.

21. BELK, W. P. and SUNDERMAN, F. W.: A Survey of the Accuracy of Chemical Analyses in Clinical Laboratories. *Am. J. Clin. Path.*, **17**:853-861 (Nov.) 1947.

22. BERLIN, R.: Primary Hyperplasia of Parathyroid Glands Associated with Ulcers in Oesophagus and Duodenum and Polycythemia of Splenomegalic Type. *Acta med. Scandinav.*, **135**:18-24, 1949.

23. BLACK, B. M.: Surgical Aspects of Hyperparathyroidism. Review of Sixty-three Cases. *Surg., Gynec. & Obst.*, **87**:172-182 (Aug.) 1948.

24. BLACK, B. M. and HAYNES, A. L.: Intrathyroid Hyperfunctioning Parathyroid Adenomas: Report of 2 Cases. *Proc. Staff Meet., Mayo Clin.*, **24**:408-413 (Aug. 3) 1949.

25. BLACK, B. M. and HAYNES, A. L.: Hyperfunctioning Carcinoma of Parathyroid Origin with Local Recurrence and Metastasis: Subsequent Report of a Case. *Proc. Staff Meet., Mayo Clin.*, **26**:309-312 (Aug. 1) 1951.

26. BLACK, B. M. and SPRAGUE, R. G.: Hyperparathyroidism Due to Diffuse Primary Hypertrophy and Hyperplasia of the Parathyroid Glands; Report of Case. *Proc. Staff Meet., Mayo Clin.*, **22**:73-80 (Feb. 19) 1947.

27. BLACK, B. M. and WATTS, C. F.: Cysts of Parathyroid Origin. Report of Two Cases and Study of Incidences and Pathogenesis of Cysts in Parathyroid Glands. *Surgery*, **25**:941-949 (June) 1949.

28. BOYD, J. D.: Development of the Thyroid and Parathyroid Glands and the Thymus. *Ann. Roy. Coll., Surgeons*, **7**:455-471 (Dec.) 1950.

29. BURNETT, C. H., COMMONS, R. R., ALBRIGHT, FULLER and HOWARD, J. E.: Hypercalcemia Without Hypercalcuria or Hypophosphatemia, Calcinosis and Renal Insufficiency; a Syndrome Following Prolonged Intake of

Milk and Alkali. *New England J. Med.*, **240**:787-794 (May 19) 1949.

30. CAMP, J. D. and OCHSNER, H. C.: The Osseous Changes in Hyperparathyroidism Associated with Parathyroid Tumor: a Roentgenologic Study. *Radiology.* **17**:63-69 (July) 1931.

31. CASTLEMAN, B. and MALLORY, T. B.: Pathology of Parathyroid Gland in Hyperparathyroidism; Study of 25 Cases. *Am. J. Path.*, **11**:1-72 (Jan.) 1935.

32. CASTLEMAN, B. and MALLORY, T. B.: Parathyroid Hyperplasia in Chronic Renal Insufficiency. *Am. J. Path.*, **13**: 553-574 (July) 1937.

33. CHURCHILL, E. D. and COPE, O.: Parathyroid Tumors Associated with Hyperparathyroidism: 11 Cases Treated by Operation. *Surg., Gynec. & Obst.*, **58**:255-271 (Feb. 15) 1934.

34. CLAGETT, O. T., EATON, L. M. and GLOVER, R. P.: Thymectomy for Myasthenia Gravis. Surgical Technique. *Surgery*, **26**:852-860 (Nov.) 1949.

35. COLLIP, J. B.: The Extraction of a Parathyroid Hormone Which Will Prevent or Control Parathyroid Tetany and Which Regulates the Level of Blood Calcium. *J. Biol. Chem.*, **63**:395-438 (Mar.) 1925.

36. COLLIP, J. B.: The Parathyroid Glands. *Medicine*, **5**:1-57 (Feb.) 1926.

37. COLLIP, J. B., CLARK, E. P. and SCOTT, J. W.: The Effect of Parathyroid Hormone on Normal Animals. *J. Biol. Chem.*, **63**:439-468 (Mar.) 1925.

38. COPE, OLIVER: Surgery of Hyperparathyroidism: The Occurrence of Parathyroids in the Anterior Mediastinum and the Division of the Operation into Two Stages. *Ann. Surg.*, **114**:706-733 (Oct.) 1941.

39. COPE, OLIVER: The Endocrine Aspect of Enlargements of the Parathyroid Glands. *Surgery*, **16**:273-288 (Aug.) 1944.

40. CRAWFORD, J. D., OSBORNE, M. M., JR., TALBOT, N. B., TERRY, MARY L. and MORRILL, MARY F.: The Para-

thyroid Glands and Phosphorus Homeostasis. *J. Clin. Investigation*, **29**:1448-1461 (Nov.) 1950.

41. DAVIES-COLLEY, N.: Bones and Kidneys from a Case of Osteomalacia in a Girl Aged 13. *Tr. Path. Soc. London*, **35**:285-297, 1884.

42. DAWSON, J. W. and STRUTHERS, J. W.: Generalised Osteitis Fibrosa with Parathyroid Tumour and Metastatic Calcification: Including a Critical Discussion of the Pathological Processes Underlying Osseous Dystrophies. *Edinburgh M. J.*, **30**:421-559 (Oct.) 1923.

43. DUKEN, J.: Beitrag zur Kenntnis der malacischen Erkrankungen des kindlichen Skelettsystems: Spätrachitis und Osteodystrophia fibrosa. *Ztschr. f. Kinderh.*, **46**:114-136, 1928.

44. ELLSWORTH, READ and FUTCHER, P. H.: The Effect of Parathyroid Extract upon Serum Calcium of Nephrectomized Dogs. *Bull. Johns Hopkins Hosp.*, **57**:91-98 (Aug.) 1935.

45. ENGFELDT, BENGT: Studies on Parathyroidal Function in Relation to Hormonal Influences and Dietetic Conditions. *Acta Endocrinol., Suppl.* **6**:1-118, 1950.

46. ERDHEIM, J.: Ueber Epithelkörperbefunde bei Osteomalacie. *Sitzungsb. d. k. Akad. d. Wissensch. Math.-naturw. Cl.*, **116**:311-370, 1907.

47. FLOCKS, R. H.: Prophylaxis and Medical Management of Calcium Urolithiasis: the Rôle of the Quantity and Precipitability of the Urinary Calcium. *J. Urol.*, **44**:183-190 (Aug.) 1940.

48. FREEMAN, L. W.: The Metabolism of Calcium in Patients with Spinal Cord Injuries. *Ann. Surg.*, **129**:177-184 (Feb.) 1949.

49. FRITZ, G. E. and BRINES, O. A.: The Cell Type of Secondary Parathyroid Hyperplasia. *Am. J. Path.*, **27**:265-275 (Mar.-Apr.) 1951.

50. GAUGELE, K.: Zur Frage der Knochencysten und der Ostitis fibrosa von Recklinghausen's. *Arch. f. klin. Chir.*, **83**:953-976, 1907.

51. Gentile, R. J., Skinner, H. L. and Ashburn, L. L.: The Parathyroid Glands; Malignant Tumor with Osteitis Fibrosa Cystica. *Surgery,* **10**:793-810 (Nov.) 1941.

52. Gilmour, J. R.: The Gross Anatomy of the Parathyroid Glands. *J. Path. & Bact.,* **46**:133-149 (Jan.) 1938.

53. Gilmour, J. R. and Martin, W. J.: The Weight of the Parathyroid Glands. *J. Path. & Bact.,* **44**:431-462 (Mar.) 1937.

54. Gley, M. E.: Sur les fonctions du corps thyroïde. *Compt. rend. Soc. de biol.,* **43**:841-847 (Dec. 19) 1891.

55. Gold, Ernst: Ueber die Bedeutung der Epithelkörpervergrösserung bei der Ostitis fibrosa generalisata Recklinghausen. *Mitt. a. d. Grenzgeb. d. Med. u. Chir.,* **41**:63-82, 1928.

56. Greenwald, Isidor and Gross, Joseph: The Effect of the Administration of a Potent Parathyroid Extract upon the Excretion of Nitrogen, Phosphorus, Calcium, and Magnesium, with Some Remarks on the Solubility of Calcium Phosphate in Serum and on the Pathogenesis of Tetany. *J. Biol. Chem.,* **66**:217-227 (Nov.) 1925.

57. Griffin, Miles, Osterberg, A. E. and Braasch, W. F.: Blood Calcium, Phosphorus and Phosphatase in Urinary Lithiasis; Parathyroid Disease as an Etiologic Factor. *J.A.M.A.,* **111**:683-685 (Aug. 20) 1938.

58. Gutman, A. B. and Gutman, Ethel B.: A Phosphorylase in Calcifying Cartilage. *Proc. Soc. Exper. Biol. & Med.,* **48**:687-691 (Dec.) 1941.

59. Gutman, A. B., Swenson, P. C. and Parsons, W. B.: The Differential Diagnosis of Hyperparathyroidism. *J.A.M.A.,* **103**:87-94 (July 14) 1934.

60. Gutman, A. B., Tyson, T. L. and Gutman, Ethel B.: Serum Calcium, Inorganic Phosphorus and Phosphatase Activity; in Hyperparathyroidism, Paget's Disease, Multiple Myeloma and Neoplastic Disease of the Bones. *Arch. Int. Med.,* **57**:379-413 (Feb.) 1936.

61. Halsted, W. S. and Evans, H. M.: The Parathyroid Glandules. Their Blood Supply, and Their Preservation

in Operation upon the Thyroid Gland. *Ann. Surg.,* **46:** 489-506 (Oct.) 1907.

62. HANES, F. M.: Hyperparathyroidism Due to Parathyroid Adenoma, with Death from Parathormone Intoxication. *Am. J. M. Sc.,* **197:**85-90 (Jan.) 1939.

63. HANNON, R. R., SHORR, E., McCLELLAN, W. S. and Du-BOIS, E. F.: A Case of Osteitis Fibrosa Cystica (Osteomalacia?) with Evidence of Hyperactivity of the Parathyroid Bodies. Metabolic Study. *J. Clin. Investigation,* **8:**215-227 (Feb.) 1930.

64. HANSON, A. M.: The Hormone of the Parathyroid Gland. *Proc. Soc. Exper. Biol. & Med.,* **22:**560-561, 1925.

65. HAYNES, A. L.: Personal communication to the author.

66. HELLSTROM, JOHN: Clinical Experiences of Twenty-one Cases of Hyperparathyroidism with Special Reference to the Prognosis Following Parathyroidectomy. *Acta chir. Scandinav.,* **100:**391-421, 1950.

67. HOFFHEINZ: Über Vergrösserungen der Epithelkörperchen bei Ostitis fibrosa und verwandten Krankheitsbildern. *Virchows Arch. f. path. Anat.,* **256:**705-735, 1925.

68. HOWARD, J. E., CAREY, R. A., RUBIN, P. S. and LEVINE, M. D.: Diagnostic Problems in Patients with Hypercalcemia. *Tr. A. Am. Physicians,* **62:**264-269, 1949.

69. HUBBARD, R. S. and WENTWORTH, J. A.: A Case of Metastatic Calcification Associated with Chronic Nephritis and Hyperplasia of the Parathyroids. *Proc. Soc. Exper. Biol. & Med.,* **18:**307-308, 1921.

70. INGALLS, T. H., DONALDSON, GORDON, and ALBRIGHT, FULLER: The Locus of Action of the Parathyroid Hormone: Experimental Studies with Parathyroid Extract on Normal and Nephrectomized Rats. *J. Clin. Investigation,* **22:**603-608 (July) 1943.

71. JACOBY, MARTIN and SCHROTH: Ueber die Einwirkung von Calcium lacticum auf einen Fall von Ostitis fibrosa mit experimentall-therapeutischen Stoffwechseluntersuchungen. *Mitt. a. d. Grenzeb. d. Med. u. Chir.,* **25:**383-390, 1912.

72. KEATING, F. R., JR.: Hyperparathyroidism. *Am. J. Ortho-dontics*, **33**:116-128 (Feb.) 1947.
73. KEATING, F. R., JR. and COOK, E. N.: The Recognition of Primary Hyperparathyroidism: an Analysis of Twenty-four Cases. *J.A.M.A.*, **129**:994-1002 (Dec. 8) 1945.
74. KEATING, F. R., JR., SPRAGUE, R. C. and POWER, M. H.: Personal communication to the author.
75. KOHN, A.: Studien über die Schilddruse. *Arch. f. mikr. Anat.*, **44**:366-422, 1894-1895.
76. LANDON, J. F.: Parathyroidectomy in Generalized Osteitis Fibrosa Cystica. Report of a Case in a Child Two and One-half Years of Age. *J. Pediat.*, **1**:544-554 (Nov.) 1932.
77. MACCALLUM, W. G.: Tumor of the Parathyroid Gland. *Bull. Johns Hopkins Hosp.*, **16**:87-89 (Mar.) 1905.
78. MANDL, F.: Klinisches und Experimentelles zur Frage der lokalisierten und generalisierten Ostitis fibrosa. (Unter besonderer Berücksichtigung der Therapie der Litzteren). *Arch. f. klin. Chir.*, **143**:1-46, 1926.
79. MANDL, F.: Zur Technik der Parathyreoidektomie bei Ostitis fibrosa auf Grund neuer Beobachtungen. *Deutsche Ztschr. f. Chir.*, **240**:362-375, 1933.
80. McLEAN, F. C.: Activated Sterols in the Treatment of Parathyroid Insufficiency; a Review. *J.A.M.A.*, **117**:609-619 (Aug. 23) 1941.
81. McLEAN, F. C. and BLOOM, W.: Calcification and Ossification; Mobilization of Bone Salt by Parathyroid Extract. *Arch. Path.*, **32**:315-335 (Sept.) 1941.
82. McLEAN, F. C. and HASTINGS, A. B.: Clinical Estimation and Significance of Calcium-ion Concentrations in the Blood. *Am. J. M. Sc.*, **189**:601-613 (May) 1935.
83. MEYER, K. A., ROSI, P. A. and RAGINS, A. B.: Carcinoma of Parathyroid Gland. *Surgery*, **6**:190-200 (Aug.) 1939.
84. NEUFELD, A. H. and COLLIP, J. B.: The Primary Action of the Parathyroid Hormone. *Endocrinology*, **30**:135-141 (Jan.) 1942.
85. NORRIS, E. H.: Collective Review; Parathyroid Adenoma;

Study of 322 Cases. *Internat. Abstr. Surg.*, **84**:1-41 (Jan.) 1947.

86. OLIVER, W. A.: Acute Hyperparathyroidism. *Lancet*, **2**:240-244 (July 29) 1939.

87. PUGH, D. G.: The Roentgenologic Diagnosis of Diseases of Bones. In Golden, Ross: *Diagnostic Roentgenology*. New York, Thomas Nelson and Sons, 1951, pp. 351-560 AQ.

88. PUGH, D. G.: Personal communication to the author.

89. VON RECKLINGHAUSEN, F. D.: *Die fibröse oder deformirende Ostitis, die Osteomalacie und die osteoplastische Carcinose in ihren gegenseitigen Beziehungen.* Festschr. Rudolf Virchow, Berlin, 1891, 89 pp.

90. RICHARDSON, E. P., AUB, J. C. and BAUER, WALTER: Parathyroidectomy in Osteomalacia. *Ann. Surg.*, **90**:730-741 (Oct.) 1929.

91. RIENHOFF, W. F., JR.: The Surgical Treatment of Hyperparathyroidism; with a Report of 27 Cases. *Tr. South. S. A.*, **61**:340-367, 1949.

92. ROBISON, ROBERT: The Possible Significance of Hexosephosphoric Esters in Ossification. *Biochem. J.*, **17**:286-293, 1923.

93. ROGERS, H. M.: Parathyroid Adenoma and Hypertrophy of the Parathyroid Glands. *J.A.M.A.*, **130**:22-28 (Jan. 5) 1946.

94. ROGERS, H. M. and KEATING, F. R., JR.: Primary Hypertrophy and Hyperplasia of the Parathyroid Glands as a Cause of Hyperparathyroidism. *Am. J. Med.*, **3**:384-401 (Oct.) 1947.

95. ROGERS, H. M., KEATING, F. R., JR., MORLOCK, C. G. and BARKER, N. W.: Primary Hypertrophy and Hyperplasia of the Parathyroid Glands Associated with Duodenal Ulcer; Report of an Additional Case with Special Reference to Metabolic, Gastrointestinal and Vascular Manifestations. *Arch. Int. Med.*, **79**:307-321 (Mar.) 1947.

96. ROGERS, H. M., WOOLNER, L. B., JOHNS, SYLVIA M. and

SPRAGUE, R. G.: Multiple Parathyroid Adenomas Associated with Islet-cell Tumors of the Pancreas. Report of Two Cases, with Necropsy Findings. *M. Clin. North America*, **29**:1141-1156 (July) 1949.

97. SANDSTROM, IVAR: Om en ny körtel hos menniskan och atskilliga daggdjur. *Upsala läkaref. förh.*, **15**:441-471, 1880.

98. SCHLAGENHAUFER, F.: Zwei Fälle von Parathyreoideatumoren. *Wien, klin. Wchnschr.*, **28**:1362, 1915.

99. SCHNEIDER, R. W. and ROBNETT, A. H.: Diagnosis of Obscure Hyperparathyroidism. *Cleveland Clin. Quart.*, **18**:66-71 (Apr.) 1951.

100. SCHRIFFRIN, M. J.: Relationship between the Parathyroid and the Gastric Glands in the Dog. *Am. J. Physiol.*, **135**:660-669 (Feb.) 1942.

101. SELYE, HANS: Mechanism of Parathyroid Hormone Action. *Arch. Path.*, **34**:625-632 (Oct.) 1942.

102. SHELLING, D. H.: *The Parathyroids in Health and in Disease*. St. Louis, C. V. Mosby Company, 1935, 335 pp.

103. SHELLING, D. H., KAJDI, LASLO and GUTH, LENORE: Calcium and Phosphorus Studies. XIV. The Effect of Repeated Doses of Parathyroid Extract on the Chemical Composition of the Blood and Urine of the Dog: An Explanation of the Cause of Death in Parathyroid Overdosage. *Endocrinology*, **22**:225-235 (Feb.) 1938.

104. SMITH, F. B. and COOKE, R. T.: Acute Fatal Hyperparathyroidism. *Lancet*, **2**:650-651 (Nov. 23) 1940.

105. THOMSON, D. L. and COLLIP, J. B.: The Parathyroid Glands. *Physiol. Rev.*, **12**:309-383 (July) 1932.

106. TWEEDY, W. R., TEMPLETON, R. D. and McJUNKIN, F. A.: The Effect of Complete Renal Insufficiency on the Action of Parathyroid Hormone in the Dog. *Am. J. Physiol.*, **115**:514-519 (May) 1936.

107. VASSALE, G. and GENERALI, F.: Fonction parathyréoïdienne et fonction thyréoïdienne. *Arch. ital. de biol.*, **33**:154-156, 1900.

108. WALTON, A. J.: The Surgical Treatment of Parathyroid Tumours. *Brit. J. Surg.*, **19**:285-291 (Oct.) 1931.

109. WELSH, D. A.: Concerning the Parathyroid Glands: A Critical, Anatomical, and Experimental Study. *J. Anat. & Physiol.*, **32**:292-307 (Jan.); 380-402 (Apr.) 1898.

110. WILDER, R. M.: Hyperparathyroidism: Tumor of the Parathyroid Glands Associated with Osteitis Fibrosa. *Endocrinology*, **13**:231-244 (May-June) 1929.

111. WILDER, R. M. and HOWELL, L. P.: Etiology and Diagnosis in Hyperparathyroidism; a Review of One Hundred and Thirty-five Proved Cases. *J.A.M.A.*, **106**:427-431 (Feb. 8) 1936.

112. WILTON, AKE: On the Genesis of "Osteitis Fibrosa Generalisata" (Engel-Recklinghausen Disease). *Acta path. et. microbiol. Scandinav.*, **23**:1-51, 1946.

INDEX

tissue calcification of, 16
Osteolytic carcinomatosis, 63
Osteolytic metastatic growths, 66
Osteomalacia, 7, 18, 62
Osteoporosis, 33, 62
Osterberg, A. E., 13, 100
Oxygen, 82

P

Paget's disease, 47, 62
Pain, 42, 51
  severe, 93
  skeletal, 93
Pancreas, tumors of islet cells of, 52
Paralysis, 62
  vocal cords, 93
Parathyroid
  adenomas, 75-81
    location of, 75-77
      anterior mediastinum, 75-76
      cervical incision, 77
      cervical region, 75
      intrathoracic goiter, 76
      mediastinum, 75-76
      posterior mediastinum, 75-76
      sternotomy incision, 76
      vascular pedicle, 76
    size, 78-81
      demineralization, 78
      generalized osteitis fibrosa, 78-79
      hypercalcemia, 78-79
      hypercalciuria, 78
      level of calcium in serum, 78-79
      negative calcium balance, 78
      osseous disease, 78-79
      serum calcium, 78-79, 81
      small tumors, 78
      weight, 78-81
  extract, 10, 51, 56
    intramuscularly, 91

intravenous, 91
  massive doses, 48
glands, 68, 70-75
  atrophic, 71-72, 90
    capsule, 72
    color, 71-72
    fatty pad, 72
    fatty stroma, 71
    parenchyma, 71
    size, 71
    subcapsular vessels, 72
    vascular pedicle, 72
  location of, 72-75
    adult gland, 74
    blood supply, 74
    cervical fascia, 74
    embryonic development, 72-74
    in the adult, 73
    inferior gland, 73
    parathymus, 73
    relation to inferior pole of thyroid, 73-74
    superior gland, 73
    thyroid gland, 75
    vascular pedicles, 74
  multiple adenomas, 20
  normal, 70-71
    anastomotic channel, 71
    arterial supply, 71
    characteristic feature, 70
    color, 70
    cysts, small, 70
    dimensions, 70
    fatty pad, 70-71
    in the newborn, 70
    reticulum of vessels, 70-71
    smooth surface, 70
    vascular pedicle, 71
    weight, 70
  number of, 72
hormone, 15, 37, 92
  diuretic effect, 37
  indirect action of pituitary on, 19

This Book

HYPERPARATHYROIDISM

By B. MARDEN BLACK, M.D.

was set, printed and bound by The Collegiate Press of Menasha, Wisconsin. The engravings were made by The Northwestern Engraving Company of Menasha, Wisconsin. The page trim size is 5½ x 8½ inches. The type page is 23 x 39 picas. The type face is Intertype Caledonia, set 11 point on 13 point. The text paper is 70-lb. White Deep Falls Enamel. The cover is Pajco Lexide, No. 25, Embossing 32, Finish TT Black.

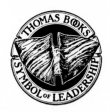

With THOMAS BOOKS *careful attention is given to all details of manufacturing and design. It is the Publisher's desire to present books that are satisfactory as to their physical qualities and artistic possibilities and appropriate for their particular use.* THOMAS BOOKS *will be true to those laws of quality that assure a good name and good will.*